P9-DEM-248

NutriSearch
COMPARATIVE GUIDE
TO
NUTRITIONAL
SUPPLEMENTS™
Consumer Edition

NutriSearch
COMPARATIVE GUIDE
TO
NUTRITIONAL
SUPPLEMENTS™

Consumer Edition

Abridged from the
NutriSearch Comparative Guide
to Nutritional Supplements,
4th (Professional) edition

by Lyle MacWilliam MSc, FP

FOR

NutriSearch Corporation

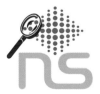

NutriSearch Comparative Guide to Nutritional Supplements™
Consumer Edition
Abridged from the *NutriSearch Comparative Guide to Nutrititional Supplements*, 4th (Professional) Edition (ISBN 978-0-9732538-6-3)

All Rights Reserved

Copyright © 2008 NutriSearch Corporation.

Published by Northern Dimensions Publishing / 2008

No part of this book may be reproduced or transmitted in any form or by any means, electronic or mechanical, including photocopying, recording or any information storage and retrieval system, without written permission from NutriSearch Corporation.

Printed and bound in the United States of America.

This guide is produced for educational and comparative purposes only. No person should use the information herein for self-diagnosis, treatment, or justification in accepting or declining any medical treatment for any health-related problems. Some medical therapies, including the use of medicines, may be affected by the use of certain nutritional supplements. Therefore, any individual with a specific health problem should seek advice by a qualified medical practitioner before starting a supplementation program. The decision whether to consume any nutritional supplement rests with the individual, in consultation with his or her medical advisor. Furthermore, nothing in this manual should be misinterpreted as medical advice.

This guide is intended to assist in sorting through the maze of nutritional supplements available in the marketplace today. It is not a product endorsement and does not make any health claim, other than to document recent findings in the scientific literature.

This guide was not commissioned by any public sector or private sector interest, or by any company whose products may be represented herein. The research, development, and findings are the sole creative effort of the author and NutriSearch Corporation, neither of whom is associated with any manufacturer or product represented in this guide.

Library and Archives Canada Cataloguing in Publication

MacWilliam, Lyle Dean
    NutriSearch comparative guide to nutritional supplements consumer edition : abridged from the NutriSearch comparative guide to nutritional supplements, 4th (professional) edition / by Lyle MacWilliam.

Includes bibliographical references.
ISBN 978-0-9732538-8-7

1. Dietary supplements. 2. Dietary supplements--Evaluation.
I. Title. II. Title: Comparative guide to nutritional supplements.

RM258 .5.M333 2008   615'.1   C2008-904892-X

To my children,
Laurie, Matthew, Tana, and Karalyn,
who make me feel blessed to be their father.

And to my wife, Arlene,
who gently leads me to knowing
that love is all there is.

DISCLAIMER

This comparative guide is intended to assist the general public in sorting through the maze of nutritional supplements available in the marketplace today. The guide does not endorse any product or manufacturer, nor does it make any health claims other than to document and summarize recent findings in the scientific literature. Those manufacturers listed in our Top-Rated Products section of the guide have been profiled in order to provide the consumer with information on leading manufacturers and their Gold Standard products. NutriSearch did not request nor did it receive remuneration from any of these manufacturers for so doing—this information is provided by NutriSearch as a public service to readers of this guide and to consumers throughout the United States and Canada.

This comparative guide was not commissioned by any public or private body, trade association, or individual company. Research and development of the guide was made possible through the combined creative efforts of NutriSearch Corporation and author, Lyle MacWilliam, MSc, FP. All costs for the publication of the guide have been borne by NutriSearch Corporation and its publisher, Northern Dimensions Publishing.

For purposes of analysis, this guide uses an independent analytical standard developed by NutriSearch Corporation. To avoid the introduction of any potential bias on the part of NutriSearch or the author, the NutriSearch Blended Standard incorporates the published recommendations of 12 independent and leading authorities in nutritional science. Using a median value of daily intakes as recommended by these authorities, the NutriSearch Blended Standard is, to our knowledge, the only independent standard currently available for comparing nutritional supplements.

This comparative guide is the intellectual property of NutriSearch Corporation. Reproduction in whole or in part by photocopy or other means is not permitted without the written consent of the author.

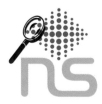

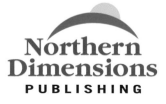

Table of Contents

Chapter 4: Medals of Achievement 4.1

Chapter 5: Top-rated Products 5.1

Chapter 6: Health Support Profiles 6.1

Chapter 7: Single Product Ratings 7.1

Chapter 8: Combination Product Ratings 8.1

Figures and Tables

I don't want to achieve immortality through my work.
I want to achieve immortality through not dying.
— *Woody Allen*

CHAPTER 1:

THE CASE FOR SUPPLEMENTATION

Insufficient vitamin intake is apparently a cause of chronic diseases. Recent evidence has shown that suboptimal levels of vitamins (below standard), even well above those causing deficiency syndromes, are risk factors for chronic diseases such as cardiovascular disease, cancer, and osteoporosis. A large portion of the general population is apparently at increased risk for this reason.

— Dr Robert Fletcher, and
Dr Kathleen Fairfield

The American Medical Association (AMA) now encourages all adults to supplement daily with a multiple vitamin. Based on a landmark review of 38 years of scientific evidence by Harvard researchers, Dr Robert Fletcher and Dr Kathleen Fairfield, the conservative *Journal of the American Medical Association (JAMA)* has rewritten its policy guidelines regarding the use of vitamin supplements. In a striking departure from its previous anti-vitamin rhetoric, *JAMA* (June 19, 2002) now recommends that, given our nutrient-poor modern diet, supplementation each day with a multiple vitamin is a prudent preventive measure against chronic disease.[1,2] The researchers point out that more than 80% of the American population does not consume anywhere near the five to eight servings of fruits and vegetables required each day for optimal health.

The *JAMA* declaration also highlights a growing concern among nutrition experts that the current recommended intakes for vitamins and minerals are too low. During World War II, the US military established the Recommended Dietary Allowances, also known as the RDAs, to prevent vitamin-deficiency disorders. In recent years, a growing volume of evidence supporting the need for higher levels of intake of many vitamins and minerals to maintain optimal health has prompted the United States and Canada to revise these recommendations; however, even the new Dietary Reference Intakes (DRIs) are based on minimal levels of nutrients, not the *optimal* levels needed to prevent degenerative diseases.

The importance of a well-balanced diet, high in fruits and vegetables, is as paramount as ever. Avoiding high-calorie, low-nutrition, over-processed, fast foods takes considerable effort, given our busy modern lifestyle. Prudence dictates that we make conscientious choices to optimize our nutritional needs. In a perfect world, all the vitamins, minerals, antioxidants, and important plant-based nutrients required to meet our daily needs would be provided in the food we eat. Today, it is necessary to fortify our diets with high-quality nutritional supplements to replenish our bodies with these missing nutrients.

Dr Robert Fletcher, co-author of the groundbreaking JAMA studies, states:

> *All of us grew up believing that if we ate a reasonable diet, that [sic] would take care of our vitamin needs. But, the new evidence, much of it in the last couple of years, is that vitamins also prevent the usual diseases we deal with every day—heart disease, cancer, osteoporosis, and birth defects.*

The diseases Fletcher mentions are not illnesses that you "catch," as you would the flu or the common cold. These are diseases of lifestyle, the consequences of years of neglect and abuse to the nutritional needs of the human body. Their onset is slow, most often completely unnoticed; but once set into motion, these disease processes unleash a cascade of harmful events that result in degeneration of the tissues and organs of the body. For this reason, they are known collectively as degenerative disease.

Degenerative Disease

While science and technology have increased our lifespan dramatically over the past few centuries, they have failed to secure for us the holy grail of long-term health. If you are part of the baby boom generation or younger, chances are very good that you will make it to that cherished centennial milestone. Chances are also very good that you will live with some form of degenerative disease that promises to rob you of the pleasure of those golden years. Ironically, it seems we have slain the dragons of infectious disease only to find that our own lifestyle has now become our mortal enemy. The sad fact is, living longer allows our dietary and lifestyle choices to *create* the circumstances of today's most common causes of death.

Degenerative diseases include today's three major killers—heart disease, cancer, and stroke. Arthritis, diabetes, osteoporosis, lupus, fibromyalgia, inflammatory bowel disorder, Alzheimer's and Parkinson's diseases are but a few of the many other forms of chronic disorders that share a common cause. Their onset is slow; their progression a process of stealth. Our bodies give little indication that we are heading down a path that will lead to cancer, heart disease, or stroke. In fact, one third of initial heart attacks are fatal. The first warning of heart disease, for these people, is their *only* warning—not much of a chance for lifestyle change.

Degenerative diseases are chronic diseases, for which there is no immediate recovery and rarely a complete cure. A degenerative disease is a life sentence, in most cases stealing years from its victims or sentencing them to a lifetime of needless suffering and pain.

In America today, over 14 million adults over the age of 65 are disabled from some form of chronic disease.[3] In fact, 80% of American seniors today suffer from at least one chronic health condition and over 50% suffer from at least two chronic conditions that seriously impede their ability to function. North of the border, more than four out of five Canadian seniors living at home suffer from one or more of the same chronic health conditions that plague their American cousins. In 1987, almost 72 out of every 100 American citizens died from a chronic degenerative disease. By 2004, 89% of deaths were caused by chronic disease—an increase of over 17% in less than less than two decades.[4, 5]

Clearly, sinister forces are at work, a reflection of our dietary and lifestyle choices that are fast tracking us toward degenerative disease.

The Roots of Degenerative Disease

Over the past several decades, scientists have attempted to ferret out the causes of degenerative disease. Unlike infectious diseases, which present a clear and present danger to the body, chronic disease processes are exceedingly subtle. Like stealth fighters, they pass beneath our radar screens until well advanced. A good example is cancer, which is often well advanced by the time it is discovered.

There is growing medical evidence that cancer and other degenerative processes initially develop through oxidative damage and through inflammatory events caused by oxidation. The fact that oxidative stress and inflammation are so closely linked to diet and lifestyle suggests that the onset of chronic disease is based on long-standing inadequacies in the nutritional status of the body that have left it vulnerable to attack.

Oxidative Stress

Back in 1954, biochemist and professor emeritus of medicine, Dr Denham Harman, proposed that disease and aging occur when cells, unprotected by proper levels of endogenous and dietary antioxidants, sustain repeated injury from an unrelenting attack of free radicals. Harman's Free Radical Theory proffered that the carnage inflicted by repeated oxidative assaults causes damage to the integrity of the cell. Like many bold scientific advances that dare to broach conventional wisdom, Harman's theory was largely ignored, even derided, until several studies in the late 1960s overwhelmingly validated his brilliant insight.

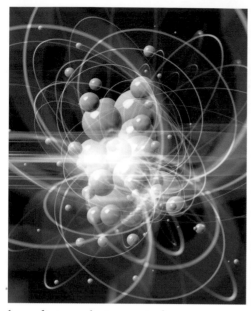

According to Harman, the cumulative damage from unchecked oxidative stress eventually destroys the molecular fidelity of the cell, impairing its function—even precipitating its death. Once tissues and organs are irreparably harmed, the stage is set for the onset of degenerative disease.

Today, most researchers believe that, collectively, degenerative diseases are simply different forms of expression of degradative events influenced by genetic endowment, environment, and lifestyle. Which disease strikes you depends as much on your individual lifestyle and lifelong dietary choices as it does on your genetic predisposition.

Systemic Inflammation

Research also shows that, beyond the immediate damage that oxidative stress invokes to the cell's molecular structures, it also kick-starts a process of systemic inflammation by activating key inflammation-promoting molecules within the cell. Nuclear factor Kappa B (NFkB) is one of several such signalling proteins activated by oxidative stress. Recent evidence shows that this protein may be the missing link between oxidation and inflammation. Once mobilized, NFkB switches on hundreds of genes that control the manufacture of numerous other cell-signalling proteins. In turn, these proteins unleash a cascade of inflammatory reactions that damage neighbouring cellular structures and lead to the onset of disease and accelerated aging. The process is silent, systemic, and deadly.

Hence, the ability to control oxidative stress and to inhibit systemic inflammation is vital to the long-term health of the cell.[6] The roles that both processes play in the manifestation of degenerative disease are discussed fully in the complete version of the *NutriSearch Comparative Guide to Nutritional Supplements, 4th (Professional) Edition.*

Preventing Degenerative Disease

The good news is that there is something we can do, regardless of our age or our health, to retard the progression of degenerative diseases. According to former US Surgeon General, Dr Everett Koop:

The preponderance of the evidence . . . substantiates an association between dietary factors and rates of chronic diseases. In particular, the evidence suggests strongly that a dietary pattern that contains excessive intake of foods high in calories, fat (especially saturated fat), cholesterol, and sodium, but that is low in complex carbohydrates and fibre, is one that contributes significantly to the high rates of major chronic diseases among Americans. It also suggests that reversing such dietary patterns should lead to a reduced incidence of these chronic diseases.[7]

The evidence clearly draws a link between our level of nutrition and our long-term health; those of us who consume a healthy diet and keep fit are likely to live longer, healthier lives. The dietary recommendations for chronic disease prevention are consistent from one specific condition to the next. In the same report mentioned above, the Surgeon General advocates a diet rich in fruits and vegetables, complex carbohydrates, and fibre. The report recommends a varied and balanced plant-based diet and warns against high-fat, calorie-dense foods that are devoid of any real nutritional value, such as those made with refined sugars and white flour.

In fact, we knew of the importance of good nutrition well before it became the focus of the US Surgeon General's report. Scientists who helped eradicate infectious diseases warned some time ago that we would be facing new health challenges based on our lifestyle choices. Most people simply accept the onset of arthritis, heart disease, and diabetes as inevitable results of the aging process—the truth is, these conditions are largely preventable.

For instance, up to 30% of heart disease can be attributed directly to obesity and oxidized cholesterol, two conditions that are lifestyle and diet related. Up to 35% of all cancer deaths, especially breast, prostate, and colon cancers, are related to diet. In 1997, the American Institute for Cancer Research and the World Cancer Fund released a report claiming that a change in diet could prevent 3 to 4 million cancer cases throughout the world each year.[8] As well, osteoporosis has been traced to diets low in calcium and vitamin D;[9] macular degeneration and cataracts arise, in part, from low intakes of antioxidants such as vitamins C and E. The pattern is undeniable.

With appropriate modifications to diet and lifestyle, 60 to 70% of the incidence of heart disease can be prevented, as can 80% of the incidence of stroke. Some experts believe that up to 80% of cancer deaths are also avoidable. As well, over 90% of type-2 diabetes, a major health risk for tens of thousands of Americans and Canadians, alike, is preventable—all through simple modifications in diet and exercise. The solution is almost too easy to imagine.

It's Your Choice

Mark Twain strikes a jocular chord when he says, "The only way to keep your health is to eat what you don't want, drink what you don't like, and do what you'd rather not." We chuckle, but, unfortunately, too many of us feel the same way.

Health is a matter of choice, such as choosing to eat a healthy balanced meal instead of a greasy burger and fries or choosing to take a brisk walk instead of watching TV. Yet, far too many of us are making poor nutrition and lifestyle choices on a consistent basis. In fact, most North Americans do it every day. If, instead, we chose to make good nutrition—including supplementation—and an active lifestyle a daily habit, we could add 5 to 15 *healthy* years to our lives. Apart from the future benefits, eating well and exercising regularly also enable us to enjoy life so much more right now!

What this Guide is About

The purpose of this guide is to provide you with a better understanding of how vitamins, minerals, antioxidants, and other plant-based nutrients—as supplements to today's inadequate diet—work together to optimize your health and reduce your lifetime risk of degenerative disease. Using an evidence-based approach, and relying on the latest research findings, this guide will show which brands of supplements will provide the most complete nutritional support to build your personal health insurance plan and help you age more gracefully.

The information in this Consumer Edition of the *NutriSearch Comparative Guide to Nutritional Supplements* is condensed from the complete version of the *NutriSearch Comparative Guide to Nutritional Supplements, 4th (Professional) Edition,* available at comparativeguide.com, amazon.com, amazon.ca and through your local bookstore.

For those readers wanting to delve even more deeply into the science of nutrition, we invite you to log on to our website at NutriSearch.ca and click on our SHOW ME THE SCIENCE section, where we discuss in greater detail the scientific evidence supporting the rating criteria used in this guide.

REFERENCES FOR CHAPTER ONE:

(1) Fairfield KM, Fletcher RH. Vitamins for chronic disease prevention in adults: scientific review. *JAMA* 2002 June 19;287(23):3116-26.

(2) Fletcher RH, Fairfield KM. Vitamins for chronic disease prevention in adults: clinical applications. *JAMA* 2002 June 19;287(23):3127-9.

(3) Wan H, Sengupta M, Velkoff VA, DeBarros KA. 65+ in the United States 2005. U S Census Bureau 2006; Available at: URL: www.census.gov. AccessedApril 14, 2006.

(4) Extracts of The Surgeon General's Report on Nutrition and Health. Washington, DC: U.S. Department of Health and Human Services; 1988.

(5) WISQARS Internet program. WISQARS Leading Causes of Death Reports, 1999 - 2004. Atlanta, GA: Office of Statistics and Programming, National Center for Injury Prevention and Control, Centers for Disease Control and Prevention; 2004.

(6) Greenwell I. The Role of Inflammation in Chronic Disease. *Life Extension Magazine* Feb. 2001. Life Extension Media.

(7) Extracts of The Surgeon General's Report on Nutrition and Health. Washington, DC: U.S. Department of Health and Human Services; 1988.

(8) Potter JD, Chavez A, Chen J et al. Food, Nutrition and the Prevention of Cancer: A Global Perspective. American Institute for Cancer Research and the World Cancer Research Fund; 1997 Sep.

(9) Reid IR. Therapy of osteoporosis: calcium, vitamin D, and exercise. *Am J Med Sci* 1996 December;312(6):278-86.

> Facts are the air of scientists.
> Without them you can never fly.
> — *Linus Pauling*
> *Nobel Laureate in Chemistry and Peace*

CHAPTER 2:

COMPARING SUPPLEMENTS

Every nutritional supplement included in this Consumers' Guide is assigned a rating based on a comprehensive analytical model developed by NutriSearch Corporation. This model is based on a compilation of the recommended daily nutritional intakes of 12 independent nutritional authorities.

Each of the 12 authorities cited has published one or more works that recommend specific daily nutritional intakes deemed important for long-term health. Each author, listed below, is acknowledged within his or her respective scientific, medical, and naturopathic field:

✔ **Robert Atkins, MD**

The late Robert Atkins was the founder and medical director of the Atkins Center for Complementary Medicine in New York City. An early proponent of the value of nutritional supplementation, Dr Atkins' best-selling book, *Dr Atkins' Vita-Nutrient Solution*, stresses the importance of daily supplementation in overcoming nutritional deficiencies found in our foods today. A practising physician and a professor of medicine at Capital University of Integrative Medicine, Dr Atkins gained recognition in 1972 with the publication of his first book, *Dr Atkins' Diet Revolution*. Subsequent to this, he wrote *Dr Atkins' Nutrition Breakthrough* and *Dr Atkins' Health Revolution*.

✔ **Phyllis Balch, CNC**

Until her death in 2004, Phyllis Balch was a leading nutritional consultant, recognized for her expertise in nutrition-based therapies. She authored several best-selling books, including: *Prescription for Dietary Wellness: Using Foods to Heal; Prescription for Herbal Healing: An Easy-to-Use A-Z Reference to Hundreds of Common Disorders and Their Herbal Remedies;* and *Prescription for Nutritional Healing: the A-to-Z Guide to Supplements,* co-authored by Dr James Balch, a certified urologist, a member of the American Medical Association, and a Fellow of the American College of Surgeons. Because of the co-authorship of *Prescription for Nutritional Healing [2002],* on which we base their recommendations, we recognize the authors as a single reference source.

✔ **Michael Colgan, PhD, CCN**

Dr Colgan is a best-selling author and internationally acclaimed speaker on anti-aging, sports nutrition, and hormonal health. His first public book, *Your Personal Vitamin Profile*, was considered a definitive guide for accurate, scientifically researched nutritional information. He has subsequently authored *Hormonal Health: Nutritional and Hormonal Strategies for Emotional Well-Being and Intellectual Longevity* and *The New Nutrition: Medicine for the Millennium*. Dr Colgan is a member of the American College of Sports Medicine, the New York Academy of Sciences, and the British Society for Nutritional Medicine. He also serves on the Council of the International and American Association of Clinical Nutritionists and the Editorial Board of the *Journal of Applied Nutrition*.

✔ **Terry Grossman, MD and Ray Kurzweil**

Dr Terry Grossman and Ray Kurzweil are co-authors of *Fantastic Voyage*, an insightful book on the science behind radical life extension. Dr Grossman is the founder and medical director of Frontier Medical Institute in Denver, Colorado. A diplomat of the American Board of Chelation Therapy (ABCT) and a member of the American Academy for Advancement of Medicine (ACAM), the International Oxidative Medicine Association (IOMA) and the American Academy of Anti-aging Medicine (A4M), Dr Grossman is a licensed homeopathic and a naturopathic medical doctor. Ray Kurzweil is one of the world's leading inventors, thinkers, and futurists. He is the author of three previous books, *The Age of Spiritual Machines; The 10% Solution for a Healthy Life;* and *The Age of Intelligent Machines*. Kurzweil received the 1999 National Medal of Technology; in 2002, he was inducted into the National Inventor Hall of Fame. Named Honorary Chairman for Innovation of the White House Conference on Small Business by President Reagan in 1986, he has received additional honours from former Presidents Clinton and Johnson.

✔ **Jane Higdon, PhD**

With over 13 years of experience as a certified family nurse practitioner, Jane Higdon also held a Master of Science in nursing, a Master of Science in exercise physiology, and a Doctorate in nutrition. Until her tragic death in 2006, Jane Higdon was a Research Associate at the Linus Pauling Institute, Oregon State University. The Linus Pauling Institute's mission is to determine the function and role of micronutrients and phytochemicals in promoting optimum health and in preventing and treating disease. The Institute conducts research to determine the role of oxidative stress and antioxidants in human health and disease.

✓ Philip Lee Miller, MD and Life Extension Foundation

Dr Miller and Life Extension Foundation (LEF) are co-authors of *The Life Extension Revolution: The New Science of Growing Older Without Aging* (2005). Dr Miller is the founder and medical director of the Los Gatos Longevity Institute. A practising physician for over 30 years, he is a diplomat of the American Board of Anti-Aging Medicine and serves on the Medical Advisory Board of LEF, the world's largest organization dedicated to the science of preventing and treating degenerative disease and aging. In addition to developing unique disease treatment protocols, LEF funds pioneering scientific research aimed at achieving an extended, healthy lifespan. At the heart of LEF's mission are its research programs for identifying and developing new therapies to slow and reverse the deterioration associated with aging.

✓ Earl Mindell, RPh, MH

Earl Mindell has written 48 books on nutrition and health, including the best-seller, *Dr Mindell's Vitamin Bible*, published in the mid 1980s. Subsequent publications include *Earl Mindell's Vitamin Bible for the 21st Century; Dr Mindell's What You Should Know About Creating Your Own Personal Health Plan; Earl Mindell's Herb Bible; Earl Mindell's Food as Medicine; Shaping up with Vitamins;* and *Earl Mindell's Anti-Aging Bible.* Mindell received a Bachelor of Science in Pharmacy in 1964, earning his Master's in Herbal Medicine in 1995. He is a registered pharmacist and a Fellow of the British Institute of Homeopathy. Mindell serves as a Director of the Corporate Board for the Illinois College of Physicians and Surgeons and is a professor of nutrition.

✓ Michael Murray, ND

Dr Murray is one of the world's leading authorities on natural medicine. He is a faculty member of Bastyr University, where he also serves on the Board of Trustees. A meticulously researched author and lecturer, Dr Murray has published more than 20 books on natural medicine, including the *Encyclopedia of Natural Medicine* and the *Encylopedia of Nutritional Supplements,* from which we base his recommendations. In addition to his private practice as a consultant to the health food industry, he has been instrumental in bringing many effective natural products to North America. Dr Murray is currently Director of Product Development and Education for Natural Factors, manufacturers of quality natural health products.

✓ Richard Passwater, PhD

Dr Passwater is a member of the American Chemical Society and a Fellow of the American Institute of Chemistry. Twice honoured by the Committee for World Health, his scientific contributions have garnered him worldwide recognition. Dr Passwater's discovery of biological antioxidant synergism in 1962 has been the focus of his research since that time. In 1973, Dr Passwater's article, *Cancer: New Directions,* was the first to report that a synergistic combination of antioxidant nutrients significantly reduces cancer incidence. Dr Passwater's pioneering work with Drs Linus Pauling and James Enstrom highlighted the protective effect of vitamin E against heart disease. His best selling book, *Supernutrition: Megavitamin Revolution,* legitimized megavitamin therapy. Dr Passwater's most recent public books include *The Antioxidants; The New Supernutrition;* and *Cancer Prevention and Nutritional Therapies.* He is the nutrition editor for *The Experts Journal of Optimal Health* and the scientific editor for *Whole Foods,* and he serves on the editorial board of the *Journal of Applied Nutrition.* Dr Passwater is also the Director of the Solgar Nutritional Research Center.

√ Nicholas Perricone, MD

Dr Perricone is a board-certified clinical and research dermatologist. An internationally recognized anti-aging expert, award-winning inventor, and a respected scientific researcher, Dr Perricone is an Adjunct Professor of Medicine at Michigan State University's College of Human Medicine. Certified by the American Board of Dermatology, he is also a Fellow of the New York Academy of Sciences, the American College of Nutrition, the American Academy of Dermatology, and the Society of Investigative Dermatology. Dr Perricone has served as Assistant Clinical Professor of Dermatology at Yale School of Medicine and as Chief of Dermatology at Connecticut's Veterans Hospital. He is author of *The Perricone Weight-loss Diet* and *The Acne Prescription* and has written three New York Times bestsellers: *The Wrinkle Cure; The Perricone Prescription;* and *The Perricone Promise.*

√ Ray Strand, MD

Dr Strand has practised family medicine for over 30 years, focussing over the past decade on nutritional medicine. An articulate advocate for the integration of optimal nutrition and advanced nutritional therapies in preventive healthcare, he is a member of the Medical Advisory Board of USANA Health Sciences. Dr Strand has lectured on nutritional medicine across the United States, Canada, Australia, New Zealand, and England. His publications include *Bionutrition: Winning the War Within; Death by Prescription; Healthy for Life; What Your Doctor Doesn't Know About Nutritional Medicine May Be Killing You; Preventing Diabetes;* and *Living by Design.*

✓ Julian Whitaker, MD

Dr Whitaker became fascinated early in his career by the preventive and healing powers of nutrition and natural therapies. Practising at the Pritikin Longevity Center subsequent to 1976, Dr Whitaker remarked, "I saw patients get well—not as a result of dangerous drugs or risky surgical procedures, but through the powerful effects of diet and exercise. And not only did these patients drop their medications, they *dropped their diseases.*" [emphasis added] Dr Whitaker was instrumental in forming the California Orthomolecular Medical Society, and in 1979 launched the Whitaker Wellness Institute Medical Clinic, where patients participate in an intensive program of diet, exercise, nutritional and herbal supplementation, and lifestyle change. Dr Whitaker is the author of several popular books, including *Reversing Diabetes; Reversing Heart Disease;* and *Dr Whitaker's Guide to Natural Healing.* Board certified in anti-aging medicine, Dr Whitaker belongs to the American College for Advancement in Medicine and is a founding member of the American Preventive Medicine Association.

In using the preceding authors' scientific insights to construct our standard, we recognize the immense contribution that they have made, individually and collectively, to the advancement of scientific knowledge and the pursuit of optimal health.

The Blended Standard

The individual recommendations for daily nutrient intakes from the 12 authorities cited above are pooled to construct the *Blended Standard*, the yardstick by which every product in this Consumer's Guide is compared. For a nutrient to qualify for inclusion in the *Blended Standard*, 3 of the 12 authorities must cite a recommended daily intake for the specified nutrient. In all, 47 nutrient categories, consisting of 19 vitamins or vitamin-like factors, 13 minerals, 5 phytonutrient complexes, 3 essential fatty acids, and 7 other nutritional factors, are identified and incorporated into the standard. The recommended daily intake for each nutrient is determined, wherever possible, by calculating the median (middle) value from those authorities who provide a specific dosage recommendation. In some cases (noted in the Legend for the Blended Standard Table on page 2.8), where recent scientific evidence has eclipsed the recommendations, NutriSearch provides a recommended daily intake—or removes a previously recommended nutrient—based upon these new findings.

With the exception of Passwater's recommendations (which are based on diet, level of health, and physical activity), the recommended daily intakes published by each author are presented for the general adult population. Passwater's lower two categories (C and D) are selected for inclusion in the *Blended*

Continued on page 2.9

TABLE 2-1: NUTRISEARCH BLENDED STANDARD

Nutritional Components	Amt	Blended Standard Median	NOTES	Upper Limits
Vitamins				**(U L)**
Vitamin A	IU	5,000		10,000 IU
Vitamin D	IU	400		2,000 IU
Vitamin K	µg	180		Undetermined
B-Complex Vitamins				
Biotin	µg	250		Undetermined
Folic Acid	µg	600		1,000 µg
Vitamin B1 (thiamin)	mg	55		Undetermined
Vitamin B2 (riboflavin)	mg	45		Undetermined
Vitamin B3 (niacin)	mg	[28]		35 mg
Vitamin B3 (niacinamide)	mg	60		Undetermined
Vitamin B5 (Pantethine)	mg	ID		Undetermined
Vitamin B5 (Pantothenic acid)	mg	75		Undetermined
Vitamin B6 (pyridoxine)	mg	63		100 mg
Vitamin B6 (pyridoxyl-5-phosphate)	mg	ID		Undetermined
Vitamin B12 (cobalamin)	µg	175		Undetermined
Antioxidant Vitamins and Nutrients				
Coenzyme Q10	mg	60		Undetermined
alpha-Lipoic acid	mg	100		Undetermined
para-Aminobenzoic acid	mg	N R		Undetermined
Vitamin C	mg	1,500		2,000 mg
Vitamin E (as alpha tocopherol)	IU	600		1,467 IU (1,000 mg)
Vitamin E (as gamma tocopherol or mixed tocopherols)	mg	200	1	Undetermined
Bioflavonoid Complex				
Bioflavonoids (mixed/citrus)	mg	540	2	Undetermined
Hesperidin	mg	ID		Undetermined
Phenolic compounds (see comment in legend)	mg	25	3	Undetermined
Pinus Epicatechins	mg	ID		Undetermined
Procyanidolic Oligomers	mg	100		Undetermined
Quercetin	mg	ID		Undetermined
Resveratrol (3,4',5-trihydroxystilbene)	mg	ID		Undetermined
Rutin	mg	ID		Undetermined
Carotenoids				
Astaxanthin (marine carotenoid)	mg	ID		
beta Carotene	IU	13,750		Undetermined
Carotenoids (mixed)	IU	5,625	4	Undetermined
Lutein/Zeaxanthin	mg	5		Undetermined
Lycopene	mg	15		Undetermined
Glutathione Complex				
acetyl-l-Cysteine	mg	76		Undetermined
Cysteine	mg	ID		Undetermined
Glutathione	mg	N R		Undetermined

continued on next page

TABLE 2-1: NutriSearch Blended Standard   2.7

continued from previous page

Lipid Metabolism				
acetyl-l-Carnitine	mg	500		Undetermined
Carnitine	mg	500		Undetermined
Choline	mg	94		3,500 mg
Inositol	mg	125		Undetermined
Lecithin	mg	350	5,6	Undetermined
alpha-Linolenic acid (an omega-3 essential fatty acid)	mg	3,125		Undetermined
conjugated Linoleic acid (CLA)	mg	ID		Undetermined
Linoleic acid (an omega-6 essential fatty acid)	mg	ID		Undetermined
gamma-Linolenic acid (GLA)	mg	ID		Undetermined
Omega-3 fish oil (EPA/ DHA)	mg	1,141		Undetermined
Phosphatidylcholine	mg	ID	5,6	Undetermined
Phosphatidylserine	mg	ID		Undetermined
Minerals				
Boron	mg	3		20 mg
Calcium	mg	800		2,500 mg
Chromium (trivalent)	µg	238		Undetermined
Copper	mg	2		10 mg
Fluorine (as fluoride)		ID		10 mg
Iodine	µg	100		1,100 µg
Iron	mg	NR	7	45 mg
Magnesium	mg	[280]	8	350 mg
Manganese	mg	7		11 mg
Molybdenum	µg	65		2,000 µg
Potassium	mg	215		Undetermined
Selenium	µg	150		400 µg
Silicon	mg	8		Undetermined
Vanadium	µg	75		Undetermined
Zinc	mg	25		40 mg
Other Nutritional Factors				
Arginine	mg	ID		Undetermined
Betaine (trimethylglycine or TMG)	mg	350		Undetermined
Bromelaine (digestive enzymes)	mg	ID		Undetermined
Carnosine	mg	1,000		Undetermined
Dimethylglycine (DMG)	mg	ID		Undetermined
Dimethylaminoethanol (DMAE)	mg	ID		Undetermined
Garlic extract (standardized)	mg	ID		Undetermined
Gingko Biloba	mg	ID		Undetermined
Glucosamine	mg	ID		Undetermined
Glutamine	mg	ID		Undetermined
Indole-3-carbinol	mg	ID		Undetermined
Lysine	mg	ID		Undetermined
Melatonin	mg	ID		Undetermined
Methionine	mg	ID		Undetermined
Octacosanol	µg	ID		Undetermined
Taurine	mg	ID		Undetermined
Tyrosine	mg	ID		Undetermined
Vinpocetine	mg	ID		Undetermined

Table of Notes for the Blended Standard (see previous pages)

Upper Limits (UL) - The upper level of intake considered safe for use by adults, incorporating a safety factor, Food and Nutrition Board of the Institute of Medicine

References by author

Balch, PA. *Prescription for Nutritional Healing*, Avery Books, New York, NY, 2002.

Colgan, M. *Hormonal Health*, Apple Publishing, Vancouver, BC, 1996.

Mindell, E. *What You Should Know about Creating Your Personal Vitamin Plan*, Keats Pub., New Canaan, CT, 1996.

Murray, M and Pizzorno J. *Encyclopedia of Natural Medicine*, Prima Publishing, Rocklin, CA, 1998.

Murray, M. *Encyclopedia of Nutritional Supplements*, Prima Publishing, Rocklin, CA, 1996.

Passwater, RA. *The New Supernutrition*, Simon and Schuster Inc. New York, NY, 1991.

Strand, R. *What Your Doctor Doesn't Know about Nutritional Medicine May Be Killing You*, Thomas Nelson Inc. Nashville TN, 2002.

Whitaker, J. *Dr. Whitaker's Guide to Natural Healing*, Prima Publishing, Rocklin CA, 1996.

Perricone, N. *The Perricone Weight-loss Diet*, Ballantine Books, New York, 2005.

Kurzweil, R and Grossman, T. *Fantastic Voyage*, Holtzbrinck Publishers, 2004.

Atkins RC. *Dr. Atkins' Vita-nutrient Solution*, Fireside Printers, New York, 1999.

Miller, PL. and the Life Extension Foundation, *The Life Extension Revolution*, Bantam Dell, New York, 2005.

Higdon J. and the Linus Pauling Institute. *An Evidence-based Approach to Vitamins and Minerals*, Thieme Publishers, New York, 2003.

Legend

1	based on the recommended 2:1 ratio of alpha tocopherol to gamma tocopherol (see Chapter 9 in the *NutriSearch Comparative Guide to Nutritional Supplements, 4th (Professional) Edition*) also see Helzlsouer KJ et al, *J Nat Canc Inst*. 2000;92(24):2018-2023
2	also includes values for hesperedin, quercetin, rutin, and pinus epicatechins
3	Level of Phenolic Acids adapted from: Visioli F et al. *Atheroclerosis* 1995, 117: 25-32.
4	Strand: conversion from mg to IU provided by Murray MT, *Encyclopedia of Nutritional Supplements*, page 25
5	Colgan: lecithin specified in form of phosphatidyl-choline
6	Passwater: 1-2 caps estimated at 1000 mg/cap as lecithin
7	Balch: only if an iron deficiency exists
8	350 mg represents the Upper Limit for a pharmacological agent only
ID	Insufficient Data
NR	Not Recommended
[#]	daily recommended intake truncated at 80% of Upper Safe Limit for that nutrient

continued from page 2.5

Standard. These categories represent individuals who have poor-to-average diets, poor-to-average health, take little or no exercise and live a sedentary lifestyle, reflecting today's general profile of the North American adult population.

The recommendations for daily intake compiled in the *Blended Standard* are used in determining appropriate levels of intake for each of the Health Support Criteria developed for the rating of each product. These 18 criteria are summarized in Chapter 3 of this guide. A more complete discussion of each criterion is available in the complete version of the *NutriSearch Comparative Guide to Nutritional Supplements,*™ *4th (Professional) Edition,* or on our website at www.NutriSearch.ca. On the homepage, click on SHOW ME THE SCIENCE, located on the left menu bar. Here, you can access a complete description of each criterion along with the relevant scientific references.

Limitations of the Study

The products reviewed in this comparison represent a vast range of nutritional options available in the marketplace today. By necessity, NutriSearch has limited the selection to include only those products that meet specified criteria.

A qualifying product:

√ must comprise a broad-spectrum nutritional supplement formulated for general preventive maintenance rather than a specified therapeutic use;

√ must contain a comprehensive assortment of both minerals and vitamins;

√ may contain assorted antioxidants and plant-based nutrients;

√ must be formulated in tablet, capsule, or liquid form and have a specified daily dosage; and

√ must provide a comprehensive list of ingredients, along with specified amounts (in μg, mg or IU) for each nutrient in the formulation.

Individual products may contain nutrients other than those listed in the *Blended Standard.* With the exception of iron,* nutrients are *not* included in the comparison if those nutrients are not identified in the *Blended Standard.* In addition, while a manufacturer may list a nutrient identified in the *Blended Standard,* the nutrient is not included in the comparison if the exact amount (μg, mg or IU) of the nutrient is not provided or cannot be determined. For example, if vitamin A in a product is shown as "5,000 IU of vitamin A with beta carotene" the entire amount is entered as vitamin A because the precise amount of beta carotene cannot be determined.

---

* Due to recent findings on its potential toxicity, we have eliminated iron as a component of the *Blended Standard*; however, because of its continued use in many supplements, iron continues to be included in the criterion for potential toxicity.

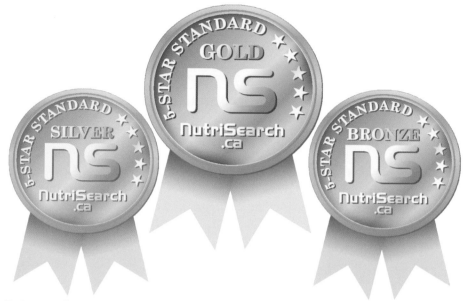

Manufacturing Quality

Our initial product rating does not consider compliance with current Good Manufacturing Practices (cGMP) nor does it include a laboratory analysis of product content. The rating is based solely on the content of the product label or monograph. However, those manufacturers with products achieving a five-star rating are invited by NutriSearch to demonstrate their commitment to quality by providing proof of their level of GMP compliance and by furnishing a notarized certificate of analysis for their product(s). This requires submission of evidence of an independent audit of current manufacturing practices and an independent laboratory analysis of product content, including identity and potency. Manufacturers who provide such standards of evidence qualify for the NutriSearch Medal of Achievement Program.™ Details of this program are discussed in Chapter 4.

Single vs. Combination Products

Many manufacturers are now selling nutritional products as packaged combinations of individual classes of nutrients. For the purpose of this comparison, we define these products as *combination products* because they consist of several individual products manufactured separately by the same company. A good example is a daily pack containing a company's foundational multiple vitamin/mineral, with an added calcium/magnesium supplement, perhaps an added phytonutrient complex (such as grape seed extract), and an added essential fatty acid capsule. While each supplement may be sold individually, they have been grouped for convenience into a daily pack. Such a product would not qualify as a *single product*, which we describe as a broad-spectrum multiple vitamin/mineral product, provided in up to two different tablets or capsules at each serving.

Comparing a combination product with a single product would not be fair because a single multiple is limited in the amounts and types of ingredients that can be included in tableted or capsule form. For example, formulating a broad-spectrum, vitamin/mineral tablet that also includes substantial amounts of essential fatty acids is problematic when it comes to issues of tableting, stability, and shelf life. Separating products into single products and combination products addresses such technical challenges. For this reason, these product classes are rated separately.

In this guide, a combination product is defined as a product that contains more than two different tablets or capsules in a single serving. Combination products are rated using the same criteria as single products; *however, the criteria for Completeness, Potency, and Inflammation also include the three essential fatty acids, EPA, DHA, and alpha-linolenic acid, which are not included in the same criteria for single products.*

The ratings for all single products and all combination products reviewed in this guide are provided in Chapters 7 and 8.

Interpreting the Graphs

Graphical comparisons are completed *only* for those products achieving a rating of four stars and above. Graphical comparisons are divided into two categories: single products and combination products. These products represent above-average products, having obtained high scores for nutritional excellence according to nutrient content and potency. These comparisons are shown in Chapter 6.

Products that display the NutriSearch Gold Medal of Achievement™ superimposed upon the graph of their *Health Support Profile*, represent the *Best of the Best*. Manufacturers of these products have gone that extra mile to verify that their products are manufactured according to pharmaceutical-model GMP. In addition, they have provided a certificate of analysis of product content, according to label, conducted by an independent third party laboratory.

The *Health Support Profile* graphs provide the consumer with a clear understanding of how a product rates in each of the 18 analytical criteria (described in Chapter 3) compiled from the *Blended Standard*. These horizontal bar graphs allow you to see the strengths of each product and identify products according to criteria that may be of particular interest to the reader (e.g. Heart Health, Liver Health, Antioxidant Support, etc.). The length of the horizontal bars in the *Health Support Profile* graph indicates whether a product's rating is *low, moderate,* or *high* for each criterion. Products that do not contain any of the appropriate nutrients for a particular health support criterion will be evident by the absence of a bar for that criterion.

There is one exception to this general description: in the criterion for Potential Toxicity, the absence of a bar indicates that there are no toxicity concerns for a product with regard to the levels of vitamin A and iron. **A red-coloured bar extending half the length (*moderate*) indicates caution regarding potential toxicity for either vitamin A or iron; a bar extending the full length (*high*), indicates caution regarding potential toxicity for *both* vitamin A and iron.**

A numerical code for each health support criterion is provided in the legend, located on pages 6.2 and 6.15. The legend makes it easy to identify a particular criterion, such as Heart Health, by matching the numerical code for the criterion in the graph with its numerical code in the legend. The intuitive nature of these graphs and their visual simplicity provide the consumer with a strong sense of relative product quality.

Qualifying the Products

All nutritional products considered for inclusion in this comparative guide are initially screened for excessive potency of specific nutrients, according to the Upper Limit of daily intake (UL) established by the US Food and Nutrition Board. The UL (shown in the right-hand column of Table 2-1 on pages 2.6 and 2.7) represents the upper level of intake for a specific nutrient deemed safe for use by adults.*

Any product containing three or more nutrients with potencies exceeding 150% of the Upper Limit is eliminated from further consideration.

The Final Product Rating (Star Rating)

Using the 18 Health Support Criteria described in Chapter 3, all qualifying products are evaluated using a series of algorithms (mathematical procedures) to arrive at a *Final Product Rating*. The development of each criterion is based on the scientific evidence available in the literature. Nutrient potencies are based on the median values of the pooled recommendations for intake established in the *Blended Standard*.

A five-star scale divided into half-star increments represents the *Final Product Rating*. A rating of five stars highlights those products possessing health support characteristics that are clearly superior to the majority of products on the market. Conversely, a rating of one star or less represents products possessing few, if any, of the health support characteristics reflected in the *Blended Standard*.

---

* The Food and Nutrition Board, Institute of Medicine, Washington, DC has recently established the ULs for a number of vitamins and minerals.

"Optimal nutrition is the Medicine of the Future."
—*Dr Linus Pauling,*
Nobel Laureate in Chemistry and Peace

CHAPTER 3:
PRODUCT RATING CRITERIA

Show Me the Science

For a more complete explanation of each criterion and the science supporting its development, the reader is referred to Chapter 9 of the complete version of the *NutriSearch Comparative Guide to Nutritional Supplements,*™ 4th (Professional) Edition. Our web site also includes the complete description of each criterion, along with the relevant scientific references. Visit us online at nutrisearch.ca.

Blended Standard

The *Blended Standard* serves as the basis for determining the *Final Product Rating* for each product. This standard, based on current nutritional science, provides a comprehensive listing of nutrients with recommended daily intakes deemed essential for

> ### AN INDEPENDENT STANDARD
>
> The NutriSearch *Blended Standard* incorporates the published recommendations of 12 independent, leading authorities in nutritional science. By using a median value of daily intakes, the *Blended Standard* avoids the introduction of any potential bias on the part of NutriSearch or the author.
>
> The weight of scientific evidence supports the need for daily levels of intake significantly higher than current recommended levels (RDAs and DRIs) for many nutrients. The NutriSearch *Blended Standard* is, to our knowledge, the only independent standard currently available for comparing nutritional supplements.

optimal health. Optimal amounts of individual nutrients in a product are based on achieving 100% of the recommended *Blended Standard* amount for that nutrient. Using this standard as the benchmark for each nutrient amount, the products are evaluated against 18 health support criteria to create a product's *Health Support Profile.*

The Health Support Profile

A five-star scale, divided into half-star increments, depicts the ranking of the *Health Support Profile* for each product. A product's score is calculated using proprietary algorithms (mathematical formulations), developed for each of the 18 health support criteria. To receive a full point for any single criterion, the product must meet or exceed the benchmark established for that criterion in the *Blended Standard*. Using a sliding scale, partial points are awarded for the partial fulfillment of each criterion. The scores are then pooled to provide a final score for each product, and the product scores are grouped so that the highest-scoring products receive five stars, and the lowest-scoring products receive zero stars. Products scoring between these extremes are grouped with similar-ranking products in half-star increments.

The last criterion, *Potential Toxicities*, penalizes the product if the formulation exceeds defined limits for those nutrients (vitamin A and iron) that demonstrate a potential cumulative toxicity.

The remainder of this chapter summarizes each criterion that comprises the *Health Support Profile* for a given product. We also provide the analytical question that addresses each criterion.

1. Completeness

The human body requires several vitamins and vitamin-like substances, a diverse group of plant-based antioxidants, numerous trace elements and minerals, and several essential fatty acids. Many of these substances can only be obtained through the diet. In all, 47 essential nutrients and nutrient categories comprise our *Blended Standard*—the definitive benchmark upon which our analysis is built. This criterion assesses whether the product contains all of the *Blended Standard* nutrients.

> *Does the product contain the full spectrum of nutrients and nutrient categories listed in the* Blended Standard *and considered essential for optimal health? To qualify, a nutrient or nutrient category must be present at a dosage that is at least 20% of the value in the* Blended Standard.

2. Potency

The potencies for the 47 essential nutrients and nutrient categories used in our *Blended Standard* reflect the need for supplementation with some nutrients at levels considerably higher than their Dietary Reference Intakes (DRIs). This criterion assesses how much of each nutrient the product contains compared to the *Blended Standard*.

> *For each nutrient in the product, what is the level of potency relative to the potency for that nutrient in the* Blended Standard?

3. Mineral Forms

Minerals are essential components of our cells. They form critical structural elements, regulate the action of nerves and muscles, maintain the cell's osmotic (water) balance, and modulate the pH (acidity) of our tissues. While minerals comprise only 4% to 5% of our total body weight, life would not be possible without them. This criterion examines mineral forms (mineral salts, chelated minerals, or organic-acid/mineral complexes), which affect the ability of the minerals to be absorbed into the blood, making them available to our cells.

For those minerals included in a formulation, how many are found in their most bioavailable forms (absorbable by the body) as amino-acid chelates or organic-acid complexes?

4. Bioactivity of Vitamin E

Natural vitamin E includes *d*-alpha tocopherol; synthetic vitamin E (commonly found in supplements as *d/l*-alpha tocopherol) is only half as effective as the natural form. This criterion assesses whether the vitamin E in a product is the natural or synthetic form.

Does the product contain the natural (d) isomer of alpha tocopherol or does the product contain the less-useful synthetic (d/l) isomers of alpha tocopherol?

5. Gamma Tocopherol

Gamma tocopherol, a type of vitamin E, possesses distinctive chemical properties that differentiate it from alpha tocopherol and may explain the observed differences in the effects of the two vitamin E forms. Studies show that gamma tocopherol reduces chronic inflammation and protects against cancers of the colon and prostate better than its alpha analogue. High-dose supplementation with alpha tocopherol alone can reduce the level of gamma tocopherol in body tissues; consequently, vitamin E supplements should contain a balance of alpha tocopherol and gamma tocopherol that is closer to what is found in nature. This criterion assesses the product for the inclusion of the gamma tocopherol form of vitamin E.

Does the product contain gamma tocopherol (or a mixture of gamma, beta, and delta tocopherols) at a potency of up to one-half the potency of alpha tocopherol in the same product? What is the potency of gamma tocopherol or mixed tocopherols in the product, compared to the potency for gamma tocopherol in the Blended Standard?

6. Antioxidant Support

The weight of scientific evidence supports supplementation with antioxidants in the prevention and treatment of many of today's common ailments. However, antioxidants do not work in isolation. For this reason, it is vital to supplement with a wide spectrum of antioxidants—an approach that is reflective of what occurs in nature. This criterion examines the nutrients that help to prevent or repair cellular damage caused by oxidation.

Does the product contain vitamin C, vitamin E (including alpha tocopherol and gamma tocopherol, or mixed tocopherols), vitamin A, beta carotene, *alpha–lipoic acid, lycopene, coenzyme Q_{10}, and selenium at potencies up to 100% of the potencies for these nutrients in the* Blended Standard?

7. Bone Health

As living tissue, healthy bones require at least 24 bone-building materials, including several vitamins, minerals, trace elements, and protein. The most important minerals are calcium, magnesium, phosphorus, and potassium; equally important is the balance between these minerals. This criterion examines the nutrients in a product that assist in bone remodelling, a process vital in warding off osteoporosis and other diseases that weaken the skeletal framework.

Does the product contain vitamin D, vitamin K, vitamin C, vitamin B_6, vitamin B_{12}, folic acid, boron, calcium, magnesium, silicon, and zinc at potencies up to 100% of the potencies for these nutrients in the Blended Standard?

8. Heart Health

Individuals with high dietary intakes of antioxidant vitamins, certain minerals, and several plant-based flavonoid compounds exhibit a lower-than-average risk of cardiovascular disease. This criterion examines several nutrients known to help protect the heart and cardiovascular system by reducing oxidative stress and suppressing inflammation.

Does the product contain vitamin E (including alpha tocopherol and gamma tocopherol, or mixed tocopherols), beta carotene, coenzyme Q_{10}, calcium, magnesium, l-carnitine or acetyl-l-carnitine, procyanidolic oligomers (PCOs), phenolic compounds, and lycopene at potencies up to 100% of the potencies for those nutrients and nutrient categories in the Blended Standard?

9. Liver Health (detoxification)

Intracellular glutathione status is a sensitive indicator of cellular health and of the cell's ability to resist toxic challenges. An important water-phase antioxidant, glutathione is one of three vital free radical scavenging mechanisms in the cell. It is also the body's pre-eminent detoxicant in the liver. While dietary glutathione is efficiently absorbed in the gut, the same is not the case for nutritional supplementation. This criterion examines those nutrients that optimize levels of glutathione and enhance liver function.

Does the product contain vitamin C, n-acetyl cysteine (including cysteine), selenium, vitamin B_2, and vitamin B_3 (including niacin and niacinamide), at potencies up to 100% of the potencies for these nutrients in the Blended Standard?

10. Metabolic Health (glucose control)

Diabetes is a chronic disorder of carbohydrate, fat, and protein metabolism. The disease begins as a constellation of metabolic changes associated with chronically high insulin levels and elevated blood-sugar levels, a condition known as *Insulin Resistance*. Conscientious dietary and lifestyle changes, including supplementation with several vitamins and minerals essential for metabolic support and the regulation of glucose metabolism can effectively reduce the risk of these disorders. This criterion examines those nutrients that help the body handle its daily sugar load, keeping systems responsive to insulin and restoring lost insulin sensitivity.

Does the product contain vitamin B_3 (including niacin and niacinamide), vitamin B_6, vitamin B_{12}, vitamin C, vitamin E (including alpha tocopherol and gamma tocopherol, or mixed tocopherols), biotin, coenzyme Q_{10}, chromium, magnesium, manganese, and zinc at potencies up to 100% of the potencies for these nutrients in the Blended Standard?

11. Ocular Health

Good eyesight and the prevention of cataracts and macular degeneration require adequate levels of several nutrients known to reduce the level of oxidative stress in the retina and lens of the eye.

Does the product contain the antioxidants, vitamin C, vitamin E (including alpha and gamma tocopherol, or mixed tocopherols), vitamin A (including beta carotene) and the carotenoids, lutein and zeaxanthin, at potencies up to 100% of the potencies for these nutrients in the Blended Standard?

12. Methylation Support

Over 40 major clinical studies confirm that high homocysteine levels are a predictive marker for heart disease, stroke, and peripheral artery disease. In fact, up to 40% of patients with heart disease express elevated levels of homocysteine. Deficiencies in certain B-complex vitamins are known to increase circulating levels of homocysteine; conversely, supplementation with these nutrients can significantly reduce circulating homocysteine by converting it to harmless methionine and cysteine. This criterion looks at those nutrients required for the body to reduce homocysteine levels in the blood.

Does the product contain vitamin B_2, vitamin B_6, vitamin B_{12}, folic acid, and trimethylglycine at potencies up to 100% of the potencies for these nutrients in the Blended Standard?

13. Lipotropic Factors

The liver and the brain are two primary targets for the accumulation of fat-soluble toxins, including pesticides and heavy metals (such as lead). Within the liver, choline and inositol assist with the elimination and removal of these noxious compounds through their ability to mobilize fats and bile. Known as *lipotropic* (fat-moving) factors, these agents have a long history of use within the naturopathic community, helping to restore and enhance liver function and treat a number of common liver ailments. This criterion examines those lipotropic agents that help the liver mobilize fats stores and remove toxins.

Does the product contain the important lipotropic (fat-moving) factors, choline or lecithin (phosphatidylcholine), and inositol at potencies up to 100% of the potencies for these nutrients in the Blended Standard?

14. Inflammation Control

Chronic inflammation, frequently induced by uncontrolled oxidative stress, is a principal mechanism by which degenerative disease takes root. Changing the balance within the body to favour the production of anti-inflammatory chemical messengers and lower the levels of inflammation is therefore an important preventive measure. This criterion examines the nutrients responsible for reducing inflammation at the cellular level, such as the omega-3 oils—particularly those found in fish oil (eicosapentaenoic and docosahexaenoic acids, or EPA and DHA) and flaxseed oil (alpha-linolenic acid).

Does the product contain eicosapentaenoic and docosahexaenoic acids, linolenic acid, gamma tocopherol, alpha-lipoic acid, vitamin C, flavonoids, procyanidolic oligomers, and the phenolic compounds from green tea, olive, and turmeric extracts, at potencies up to 100% of the potencies for these nutrients or nutrient categories in the Blended Standard?

[Due to the technical challenges, including tableting, stability, and shelf-life involved in the addition of high levels of essential fatty acids (fish oils and plant seed oils) in tableted products, the levels of these nutrient categories are only included in the Inflammation criterion for those products categorized as Combination Products.]

15. Glycation Control

Aging—the outcome of the conflict between chemistry and biology in living systems—introduces chronic, cumulative chemical modifications that compromise the structure and function of proteins and other important biomolecules within our cells. We now know that changes to these molecular structures, driven by unrelenting oxidative stress, can render them dysfunctional—a process known as glycation. Their accumulation, the detritus of an ongoing oxidative war within the cell, is a hallmark of the aging process. This criterion examines those nutrients that help slow the progress of glycation.

Does the product contain l-carnosine, vitamin E (including alpha tocopherol and gamma tocopherol, or mixed tocopherols), vitamin C, and alpha-lipoic acid at potencies up to 100% of the potencies for those nutrients or nutrient categories listed in the Blended Standard*?*

[While carnosine is available in the US market, it is restricted in products manufactured for the Canadian market. Regardless of this, our Health Support criteria are evidence-based and do not consider the regulatory question. Consequently, we have included carnosine as a critical component of our Glycation Control criterion. We recognize that this places Canadian products at a very slight disadvantage in the final product rankings. It is hoped that Health Canada will allow this important anti-aging nutrient to be made available in Canada in the near future.]

16. Bioflavonoid Profile

The flavonoids are known as "nature's biological response modifiers" because of their ability to alter the body's reactions to allergens, viruses and carcinogens, and to protect cellular tissues against oxidative attack. Flavonoids, found in the edible pulp of many fruits and vegetables, impart a bitter taste when isolated. Citrus fruits, such as oranges, lemons, limes, grapefruit, and kiwi, are particularly rich sources of flavonoids. This criterion examines the bioflavonoid family of nutrients, which works throughout the body to attack free radicals, suppress inflammation, and support many bodily functions.

Does the product contain a mixture of bioflavonoids (citrus flavonoids, soy isoflavones, quercetin, quercitrin, hesperidin, rutin, bilberry, and assorted berry extracts) and PCOs (including resveratrol, grape seed, and pine bark extracts) at potencies up to 100% of the recommended potencies for mixed bioflavonoids and PCOs in the Blended Standard?

17. Phenolic Compounds Profile

The weight of scientific evidence supporting the health benefits of polyphenols is immense. They are powerful free radical antagonists, recognized for their ability to reduce cardiovascular disease and cancer, and they demonstrate potent anti-inflammatory, anti-viral, anti-bacterial, anti-allergic, anti-hemorrhagic, and immuno-enhancing properties. The most intensely studied of the phenolic compounds include those isolated from: turmeric, a perennial herb of the ginger family and a major ingredient in curry; green tea, a rich source of compounds called catechins; and extracts from the fruit of the olive tree. This criterion examines these specific phenolic compounds, known to be exceptionally potent free radical antagonists.

Does the product contain phenolic compounds (polyphenolic acids and their derivatives, which include olive, curcumin, and the green tea extracts) at the potency for this nutrient category established in the Blended Standard?

Figure 3.1: Eighteen Important Health Support Criteria

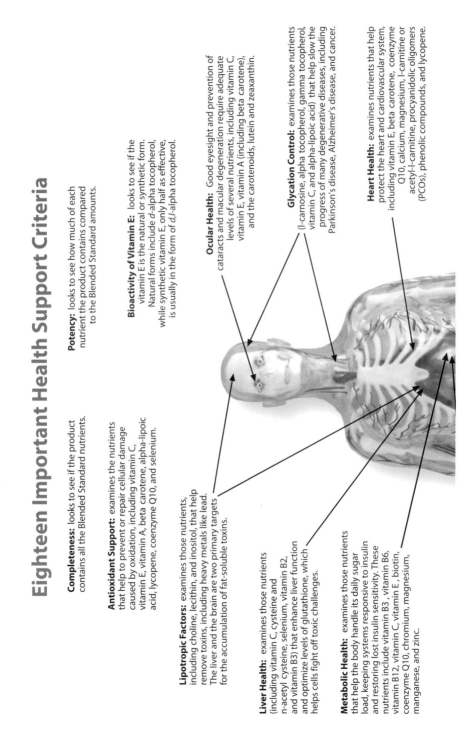

Eighteen Important Health Support Criteria

Completeness: looks to see if the product contains all the Blended Standard nutrients.

Potency: looks to see how much of each nutrient the product contains compared to the Blended Standard amounts.

Antioxidant Support: examines the nutrients that help to prevent or repair cellular damage caused by oxidation, including vitamin C, vitamin E, vitamin A, beta carotene, alpha-lipoic acid, lycopene, coenzyme Q10, and selenium.

Bioactivity of Vitamin E: looks to see if the vitamin E is the natural or synthetic form. Natural forms include *d*-alpha tocopherol, while synthetic vitamin E, only half as effective, is usually in the form of *d,l*-alpha tocopherol.

Lipotropic Factors: examines those nutrients, including choline, lecithin, and inositol, that help remove toxins, including heavy metals like lead. The liver and the brain are two primary targets for the accumulation of fat-soluble toxins.

Ocular Health: Good eyesight and prevention of cataracts and macular degeneration require adequate levels of several nutrients, including vitamin C, vitamin E, vitamin A (including beta carotene), and the carotenoids, lutein and zeaxanthin.

Liver Health: examines those nutrients (including vitamin C, cysteine and n-acetyl cysteine, selenium, vitamin B2, and vitamin B3) that enhance liver function and optimize levels of glutathione, which helps cells fight off toxic challenges.

Glycation Control: examines those nutrients (l-carnosine, alpha tocopherol, gamma tocopherol, vitamin C, and alpha-lipoic acid) that help slow the progress of many degenerative diseases, including Parkinson's disease, Alzheimer's disease, and cancer.

Metabolic Health: examines those nutrients that help the body handle its daily sugar load, keeping systems responsive to insulin and restoring lost insulin sensitivity. These nutrients include vitamin B3, vitamin B6, vitamin B12, vitamin C, vitamin E, biotin, coenzyme Q10, chromium, magnesium, manganese, and zinc.

Heart Health: examines nutrients that help protect the heart and cardiovascular system, including vitamin E, beta carotene, coenzyme Q10, calcium, magnesium, l-carnitine or acetyl-l-carnitine, procyanidolic oligomers (PCOs), phenolic compounds, and lycopene.

Figure 3.1: Eighteen Important Health Support Criteria (continued)

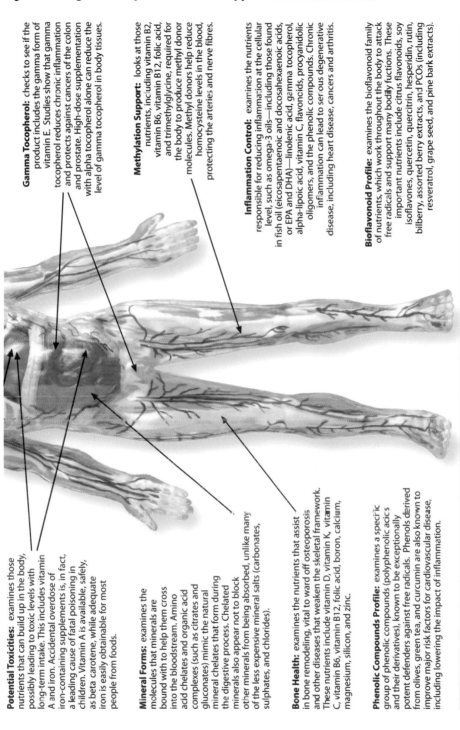

Gamma Tocopherol: checks to see if the product includes the gamma form of vitamin E. Studies show that gamma tocopherol reduces chronic inflammation and protects against cancers of the colon and prostate. High-dose supplementation with alpha tocopherol alone can reduce the level of gamma tocopherol in body tissues.

Methylation Support: looks at those nutrients, including vitamin B2, vitamin B6, vitamin B12, folic acid, and trimethylglycine, required for the body to produce methyl donor molecules. Methyl donors help reduce homocysteine levels in the blood, protecting the arteries and nerve fibres.

Inflammation Control: examines the nutrients responsible for reducing inflammation at the cellular level, such as omega-3 oils—including those found in fish oil (eicosapentaenoic and docosahexaenoic acids, or EPA and DHA)—linolenic acid, gamma tocopherol, alpha-lipoic acid, vitamin C, flavoncids, procyanidolic oligomers, and the phenolic compounds. Chronic inflammation can lead to ser ous degenerative disease, including heart disease, cancers and arthritis.

Bioflavonoid Profile: examines the bioflavonoid family of nutrients, which work throughout the body to attack free radicals and support many bodily fuctions. These important nutrients include citrus flavonoids, soy isoflavones, quercitrin, quercetin, hesperidin, rutin, bilberry, assorted berry extracts, and PCOs (including resveratrol, grape seed, and pine bark extracts).

Potential Toxicities: examines those nutrients that can build up in the body, possibly leading to toxic levels with long-term intake. This includes vitamin A and iron. Accidental overdose of iron-containing supplements is, in fact, a leading cause of fatal poisoning in children. Vitamin A is available, safely, as beta carotene, while adequate iron is easily obtainable for most people from foods.

Mineral Forms: examines the molecules that minerals are bound with to help them cross into the bloodstream. Amino acid chelates and organic acid complexes (such as citrates and gluconates) mimic the natural mineral chelates that form during the digestive process. Chelated minerals also appear not to block other minerals from being absorbed, unlike many of the less expensive mineral salts (carbonates, sulphates, and chlorides).

Bone Health: examines the nutrients that assist in bone remodeling, vital to ward off osteoporosis and other diseases that weaken the skeletal framework. These nutrients include vitamin D, vitamin K, vitamin C, vitamin B6, vitamin B12, folic acid, boron, calcium, magnesium, silicon, and zinc.

Phenolic Compounds Profile: examines a specific group of phenolic compounds (polyphenolic acids and their derivatives), known to be exceptionally potent defenders against free radicals. Phenols derived from olives, green tea, and curcumin are also known to improve major risk factors for cardiovascular disease, including lowering the impact of inflammation.

18. Potential Toxicities

In order to optimize its preventive benefits, the strategy of nutritional supplementation is to encourage long-term use. Consequently, there exists a potential risk for consumers with regard to the cumulative toxicity of particular nutrients. Most nutrients used in nutritional supplements have a high degree of safety; however, some nutrients require a degree of prudence when it comes to long-term use. Both iron and vitamin A (retinol) can become toxic when taken in high doses over a long period. Accidental overdose of iron-containing supplements is, in fact, a leading cause of fatal poisoning in children, and too much vitamin A during pregnancy can cause birth defects. Vitamin A is available, safely, as beta carotene, while adequate iron is easily obtained, for most people, from a variety of foods. This criterion examines the levels of preformed vitamin A (retinol) and iron in the product and penalizes the product rating if it contains too much of either nutrient.

> *Does the product contain vitamin A and iron (which is no longer included in the* Blended Standard*)? Does the potency of vitamin A exceed 100% of the potency for that nutrient in the* Blended Standard*? Does the potency of iron exceed 5 mg/day?*

Summary

From the 18 criteria listed in this chapter, a *Final Product Rating*, based on a five-star scale, is determined. A five-star rating highlights those products whose characteristics for optimal nutrition are clearly superior to the majority of products on the market and that approach, meet, or exceed the pooled recommendations of the *Blended Standard*. Conversely, a one-star rating or less represents products possessing few, if any, of the characteristics for optimal nutrition reflected in the *Blended Standard*. We believe that this five-star scale, divisible in half-star increments, provides an intuitive means by which the consumer can compare products based on content.

For a more complete explanation of each criterion and the science supporting its development, the reader is referred to Chapter 9 of the complete version of the *NutriSearch Comparative Guide to Nutritional Supplements,*™ *4th (Professional) Edition*, or to our website at www.NutriSearch.ca.

Quality means doing it right when no one is looking.
— Henry Ford (1863 – 1947)

CHAPTER 4:

MEDALS OF ACHIEVEMENT

Whether talking about drugs or nutritional supplements, the use of accepted standards of manufacturing (GMP) and laboratory verification of the finished product are the consumer's best assurances of quality and safety. These assurances are provided by federal regulations that govern the manufacture and sale of all natural health products—regulations that can differ markedly from country to country.

The Government of Canada requires that all manufacturers of natural health products (NHPs)* sold in Canada comply with federally mandated manufacturing and quality standards. Unlike Canada, where compliance with tough standards for the manufacturing of nutritional supplements is mandatory, in the United States compliance with pharmaceutical-level manufacturing and quality standards is entirely voluntary. It is up to the manufacturer, not any government agency, to determine if their products are safe. The US Food and Drug Authority (FDA) only investigates products *after* problems are found.

Simply put, it's a case of "buyer beware!"

Assessing Product Quality

How a nutritional product is made—what's in it and what's not *supposed* to be in it—is critical to the quality and safety of the finished product. That is why NutriSearch has introduced a new level of product assessment, called the *NutriSearch Medal of Achievement Program™* that looks beyond product content and investigates how a product is manufactured (level of GMP compliance). Through independent laboratory testing, we also look at what is actually in the finished product.

This higher standard of evidence incurs considerable cost and effort on the part of the selected manufacturers; consequently, we have offered it only to those manufacturers whose products merit a five-star rating based upon our initial analysis. The assessment is voluntary and the expense for GMP audits and laboratory testing is borne by each individual manufacturer.

Products that achieve a five-star *Final Product Rating* are eligible to participate in the **NutriSearch Medal of Achievement Program,**™ which awards

---

* In Canada, vitamins, minerals, and herbal products are commonly known as natural health products (NHPs) or *nutritional* supplements. Conversely, in the United States, such products are commonly known as *dietary* supplements.

GOLD, SILVER, or BRONZE medals based on an assessment of the level of GMP, and on third-party laboratory verification of the product's formulation.

Those manufacturers who successfully complete the program of their choice and provide proof of their level of GMP compliance qualify for either the BRONZE or SILVER Medal of Achievement. To qualify for the NutriSearch GOLD Medal of Achievement, the manufacturer must also furnish laboratory verification of the product's content according to the claims made on the product label.

Certification and Analysis Programs

Currently, there are three independent, non-government programs available in North America for the evaluation of manufacturing standards for nutritional supplements. Each program has its own level of GMP compliance, ranging from food-grade to pharmaceutical-grade:

- NPA GMP Certification Program
- NSF International Dietary Supplement Verification Program
- USP Dietary Supplement Verification Program

NutriSearch accepts certification from these programs as evidence of a manufacturer's level of GMP compliance. NutriSearch also accepts certification by Health Canada's NHPD and Australia's Therapeutic Goods Authority (TGA) as evidence of compliance with pharmaceutical-model GMPs.

Evaluation of the contents of the product is an important requirement for those manufacturers seeking the NutriSearch GOLD Medal status as a Top-Rated product. To qualify, a manufacturer must provide a certificate of analysis from a recognized laboratory. This certificate must indicate nutrient identity and content for the full range of nutrients in the product.

NutriSearch accepts the results of product analyses conducted by the NSF International Dietary Supplement Verification Program, the USP Dietary Supplement Verification Program, and independent ISO 17025 certified laboratories as proof of finished product quality.

Summary

Together, GMP certification and laboratory analysis demonstrate that the product meets recognized standards for manufacturing safety and product quality. Most importantly, it is the consumer's assurance that **"what is on the label is really in the bottle."**

For a complete description of our *NutriSearch Medals of Achievement Program*, please see the complete edition of the *NutriSearch Comparative Guide to Nutritional Supplements, 4th (Professional) Edition*, or visit our website at: http://www.nutrisearch.ca

> The preservation of health is a duty. Few seem con-
> scious that there is such a thing as physical morality.
> — *Herbert Spencer (1820-1903)*

CHAPTER 5:

TOP-RATED PRODUCTS

Over 1,600 Compared

In conducting the research for the *NutriSearch Comparative Guide to Nutritional Supplements, 4th (Professional) Edition*, we examined over 2,000 nutritional supplements throughout the United States and Canada. From this, 1,612 products qualified as multiple vitamin/mineral supplements, representing 394 manufacturers. Twenty-one of these products were eliminated because they exceeded the Upper Limits of safety for three or more nutrients. The remaining 1,591 products were further evaluated using the *Blended Standard* (described in Chapter 2) and the *product rating criteria* (described in Chapter 3).

Graphical comparisons are completed only for those products awarded four stars and above. Graphical comparisons are divided into two categories: *single* products and *combination* products. These products represent above-average products, having obtained high scores for nutritional excellence according to nutrient content and potency. The comparisons are shown in the following chapter.

Of the 1,433 single products evaluated in this guide, the products of only four manufacturers, representing a miniscule 0.6% of those evaluated, were awarded the *NutriSearch Gold Medal of Achievement.*™ Of the 179 combination products, the products of only three manufacturers, representing 3.3% of those evaluated, were awarded the *NutriSearch Gold Medal of Achievement.*™

Going for the Gold

To reach a five-star *Final Product Rating* is a significant accomplishment for a nutritional manufacturer; however, it does not tell the whole story. With any dietary supplement, the single most important factor is quality: quality research, quality formulations, and quality manufacturing. These considerations are, in turn, a reflection of the quality-control practices (GMP) employed in a product's manufacture and in the testing and verification of identity, potency, and purity of ingredients, right from the raw materials to the finished goods.

Headlining each list in Tables 5-1 and 5-2 are those select few products that have earned the *NutriSearch Gold Medal of Achievement.*™ These award-winning products represent the "Best of the Best." Not only have they attained a five-star rating according to our analytical criteria, each manufacturer has

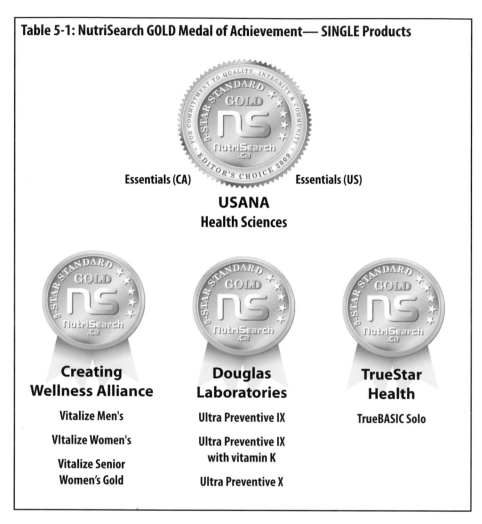

Table 5-1: NutriSearch GOLD Medal of Achievement— SINGLE Products

Essentials (CA)   Essentials (US)

USANA
Health Sciences

Creating Wellness Alliance	**Douglas Laboratories**	**TrueStar Health**
Vitalize Men's	Ultra Preventive IX	TrueBASIC Solo
VItalize Women's	Ultra Preventive IX with vitamin K	
Vitalize Senior Women's Gold	Ultra Preventive X	

demonstrated cGMP compliance and has verified through independent laboratory testing that "what is on the label is really in the bottle." These products also display the *NutriSearch GOLD Medal of Achievement*™ superimposed upon the graph of their *Health Support Profile,* provided in Chapter 6.

All products are listed alphabetically, along with their star rating, in Chapters 7 and 8. For a complete description of our *NutriSearch Medal of Achievement Program,*™ see the complete edition of the *NutriSearch Comparative Guide to Nutritional Supplements,*™ *4th (Professional) Edition*, or visit our web site at www.nutrisearch.ca.

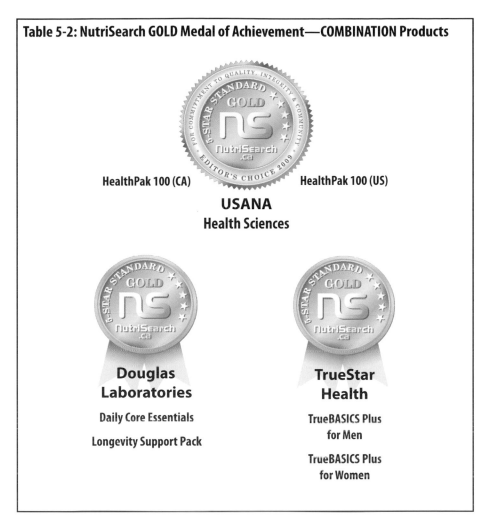

Table 5-2: NutriSearch GOLD Medal of Achievement—COMBINATION Products

HealthPak 100 (CA)   HealthPak 100 (US)

USANA
Health Sciences

Douglas Laboratories

Daily Core Essentials

Longevity Support Pack

TrueStar Health

TrueBASICS Plus for Men

TrueBASICS Plus for Women

Editor's Choice Award

Producing a Top-Rated product, according to the science-based criteria set out in the *Comparative Guide to Nutritional Supplements*, is proof of a company's commitment to product quality. However, there are several non-scientific factors that, taken together, exemplify leadership in the industry and commitment to both consumer and community.

As an added feature in this and future editions of the *Comparative Guide*, we profile one of our Top-Rated manufacturers through our *Editor's Choice Award*. This award steps beyond the science-based criteria of product formulations and looks at the company in its public role as a Corporate Good Citizen. Excellence in product quality and excellence in corporate citizenship, taken together, provide the consumer with tangible assurance of quality, integrity, and leadership.

"Excellence is an art won by training

and habituation. We do not act rightly

because we have virtue or excellence,

but we rather have those

because we have acted rightly.

We are what we repeatedly do.

Excellence, then,

is not an act but a habit."

—Aristotle (384 BC–322 BC)

Philosopher, Scientist and Physician

USANA Health Sciences

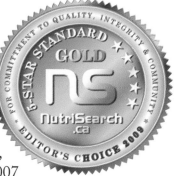

USANA Health Sciences Inc., a manufacturer of high quality nutritional and personal care products, is awarded the 2009 NutriSearch Editor's Choice Award for nutritional manufacturers. The company was founded in 1992 by Dr Myron Wentz, a noted pioneer in cellular nutrition and 2007

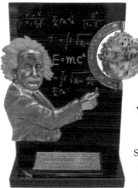

recipient of the Albert Einstein Award for Outstanding Achievement in the Life Sciences. USANA's mission is to provide the highest quality health products based on proven science. USANA products are distributed by a sales force of independent Associates around the world.

USANA products are manufactured in its own state-of-the-art facility, which is registered with the FDA as a pharmaceutical manufacturer. The company voluntarily follows Good Manufacturing Practices (GMP) for pharmaceuticals as the basis for its quality assurance program, meaning USANA treats nutritional supplements with the same care that goes into the manufacturing of pharmaceuticals. To ensure safety and consistency, USANA products are tested at every stage of the manufacturing process to meet precise quality standards.

The company's manufacturing facility has been certified to be in compliance with:

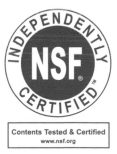

Contents Tested & Certified
www.nsf.org

- NSF International dietary supplement GMP requirements set forth in NSF/ANSI Standard 173-2006, including finished product testing
- Australia's Therapeutic Goods Administration
- Canada's Natural Health Products Directorate

As an Australian suppler, USANA's Essentials™ and HealthPak 100™ have been evaluated and approved by the Therapeutic Goods Administration to ensure they meet GMP standards for listed medicines. USANA products have also been evaluated and approved by ConsumerLab.com, a leading provider of independent test

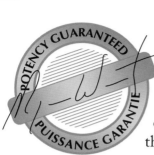

results for dietary supplements. Guaranteed to meet United States Pharmacopoeia (USP) specifications for quality, potency, and disintegration, every supplement produced by the company carries a potency guarantee which ensures that what is on the label is actually in the bottle.

To backstop its quality assurance claim, USANA pioneered an elite athlete guarantee that will compensate an athlete up to $1 million should that athlete test positive for any substance banned by the World Anti-Doping Agency as a result of taking USANA nutritional products.

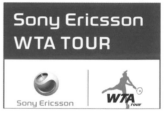

USANA is the official health supplement supplier to many world-class athletic teams, including the USA and Canada speed skating teams, Mexico's Pachuca soccer club, and the Sony Ericsson WTA Tour. USANA® supplements have been tested and found free of prohibited substances by HFL Sport Science, the testing lab for Informed-Choice and Informed-Sport, and they are also approved to carry NSF's trusted Certified for Sport™ Mark.

Honouring the values of integrity, excellence, and community, USANA has demonstrated a strong commitment to improving the lives of people at home and abroad. Employees at the company's home

In support of

CHILDREN'S HUNGER FUND®

"Serving children in need...across America and around the world."

office raise funds and devote time to tutoring local middle school students. Globally, the company and its independent Associates have donated over $6 million in cash and supplements to Children's Hunger Fund, a charity serving needy children and families worldwide.

The company enthusiastically works on behalf of its employees to create a positive work environment and support community-based health and wellness initiatives. In recognition of these efforts, USANA has repeatedly been named one of the "Best Companies to Work For" in the state of Utah and honored for its outstanding wellness programs.

As part of the global community, USANA practices responsible environmental stewardship. In 2006, the company established itself as a role model for operating an environmentally responsible business. As part of this initiative, USANA implemented a comprehensive environmental management system and became a founding reporter of the Climate Registry by voluntarily monitoring and reporting emissions.

Ranked #5 as "One of the Best 200 Small Companies in America" by Forbes magazine in 2005 and as a top revenue growth company by Mountain West Capital Network in 2007 and 2008, USANA (NASDAQ: USNA) is increasingly recognized as an innovative leader in the nutritional and direct sales industries. The company looks forward to future growth as it expands into additional international markets.

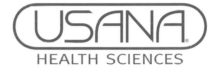

Nutritionals You Can Trust™

3838 W. Parkway Blvd.,
Salt Lake City, Utah 84120

Phone: 801-954-7100
Order Line: 888-950-9595
Web site: www.usana.com

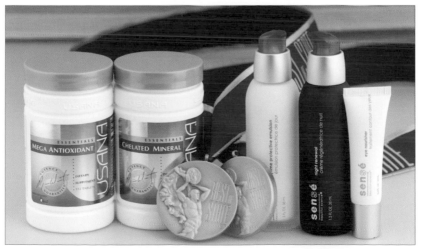

<u>GOLD MEDAL RECIPIENT:</u>

Creating Wellness Alliance

Creating Wellness Alliance (CWA), an international alliance of chiropractic professionals, offers a select line of quality nutritional products. The company prides itself in consistently maintaining the highest standards in the industry through compliance with NSF Good Manufacturing Practices (GMP) and all relevant USP certifications. The company employs a 3rd party manufacturing facility that is certified to be in compliance with:

- NSF International dietary supplement GMP requirements, including finished product testing
- Canada's Natural Health Products Directorate (NHPD)
- the US-based Natural Products Association (NPA)
- Australia's Therapeutic Goods Authority (TGA)

As dietary supplements for the Australian market must be manufactured to pharmaceutical standards, TGA approval is the ultimate confirmation of superior quality. Analytical, chemical and physical testing is performed on all nutrients by an on-site quality control/quality assurance department. CWA products are independently tested for nutrient potency and meet requirements for Kosher certification (all major authorities).

CWA has created a substantial wellness brand by developing "Best-of-Class" wellness products and offering a comprehensive lifestyle program called the Creating Wellness System. The Creating Wellness System is offered through affiliated Creating Wellness Centres operating in the United States, Canada, and New Zealand.

CWA also offers customized wellness programs for corporations, governmental bodies, and other organizations that wish to develop a culture of wellness amongst their workforce. Creating Wellness Corporate Wellness Programs provide employees with a proven method to improve their lifestyle, based on their personal goals and their current condition of health.

Product Availability: CWA products are sold through healthcare professionals at participating CWA-certified chiropractic clinics.

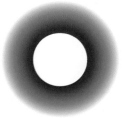

Contact Information:
Creating Wellness Alliance
Suite 750, One International Blvd
Mahwah, NJ 07495
(888) 589-WELL (9355)
www.creatingwellness.com

GOLD MEDAL RECIPIENT:

Douglas Laboratories

Douglas Laboratories is part of Atrium Biotechnologies Inc., an international company and global leader in the development, manufacturing, and marketing of dietary supplements, specialty fine chemicals, and active cosmetic ingredients. At the center of an advanced global network of specialty manufacturing, Douglas Laboratories has become a world leader in the development of scientifically based nutritional products, offering a broad selection of over 700 quality supplements.

The company regularly undertakes clinical trials designed to validate the efficacy of its products and provides custom formulations, private labeling, and packaging for customers wishing to market their own brand of supplements. All products are manufactured to stringent specifications in ISO 9001 and ISO 17025 accredited laboratories.

These laboratories meet:

- current Good Manufacturing Practices (cGMP) in accordance with USP 30
- NSF International dietary supplement GMP requirements
- GMP standards in the European Union, Australia (TGA), and Canada (NHPD)
- compliance with the Public Health Security and Bioterrorism Preparedness and Response Act of 2002, ensuring safety of all raw materials
- VCP (Vendor Certification Program) assurances of product safety and quality

Douglas Labs products meet and exceed USP standards. Written procedures for each aspect of production adhere to strict quality controls, including detailed records for each product component. Testing and sampling of all raw materials is conducted on every product batch. Microbial testing on all products ensures that they surpass microbial limit standards.

Product Availability: Douglas Labs products are available through healthcare professionals and sold through private label.

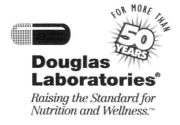

Douglas Laboratories®
Raising the Standard for Nutrition and Wellness.™

Contact Information:
Douglas Laboratories
600 Boyce Road
Pittsburg, PA 15205
888-DOUGLAB or 800-245-4440
www.douglaslabs.com

GOLD MEDAL RECIPIENT:

Truestar Health

Founded in 2001, Truestar Health embraces a comprehensive approach to optimal wellness that pinpoints five key areas of health: vitamins, nutrition, exercise, sleep and attitude. By teaching each person to balance these priorities, Truestar Health's mission is to help men, women, and children attain and maintain their healthy lifestyle goals.

To complement their treatment philosophy, Truestar Health developed the Truestar Professional Series vitamins and supplements. Formulated by a team of naturopathic and medical doctors, Truestar Professional Series supplements are designed to work synergistically for optimal results. All Truestar Professional Series supplements are manufactured to stringent specifications in ISO 9001 and ISO 17025 accredited laboratories.

These laboratories meet:

- current Good Manufacturing Practices (cGMP) in accordance with USP 30
- NSF International dietary supplement GMP requirements
- GMP standards in the European Union, Australia (TGA), and Canada (NHPD)
- compliance with the Public Health Security and Bioterrorism Preparedness and Response Act of 2002, ensuring safety of all raw materials
- VCP (Vendor Certification Program) assurances of product safety and quality

Truestar Health products meet and exceed USP standards. Written procedures for each aspect of production adhere to strict quality controls, including detailed records for each product component. Testing and sampling of all raw materials is conducted on every product batch. Microbial testing on all products ensures that they surpass microbial limit standards.

Product Availability: Truestar products are sold online and through Truestar health and fitness centres located throughout Canada.

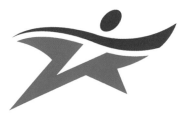

Contact Information:
Truestar Health
55 St. Clair Ave W.
Toronto, Canada
1 888 448 TRUE (8783)
www.truestar.com

"Vitamins, if properly understood and applied, will help
us to reduce human suffering to an extent which the
most fantastic human mind would fail to imagine."
—*Albert Szent-Györgyi (1893-1986)*
Nobel Laureate in Physiology and Medicine

CHAPTER 6:

HEALTH SUPPORT
PROFILES

This section provides the reader with
a graphical look at all of the
Four- and Five-Star-Rated Products.

*To be included in the graphs, products must attain a Final Product Rating
of four stars or above. Each qualifying manufacturer's highest-rated product
in each of the US and Canadian markets is graphically displayed using our
18* Health Support Profile *criteria, which rank the product according to an
incremental five-star scale.*

*Where gender-specific products of the same manufacturer attain four stars or
above, both products are graphically displayed. Those products demonstrating
compliance with pharmaceutical-model Good Manufacturing Practices and
laboratory verification of contents and purity are designated with the* NutriSearch GOLD Medal of Achievement.™

Health Support Profile Legend

1. Completeness
2. Potency
3. Mineral Forms
4. Bioactivity of Vitamin E
5. Gamma Tocopherol
6. Antioxidant Support
7. Bone Health
8. Heart Health
9. Liver Health
10. Metabolic Health
11. Ocular Health
12. Methylation Support
13. Lipotropic Factors
14. Inflammation Control
15. Glycation Control
16. Bioflavonoid Profile
17. Phenolic Compounds
18. Potential Toxicities

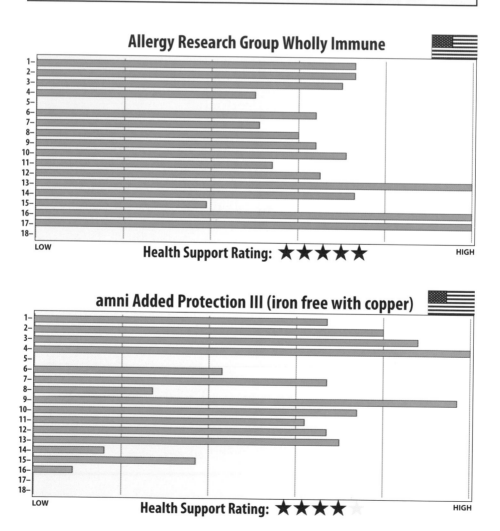

Allergy Research Group Wholly Immune

LOW — HIGH

Health Support Rating: ★★★★★

amni Added Protection III (iron free with copper)

LOW — HIGH

Health Support Rating: ★★★★☆

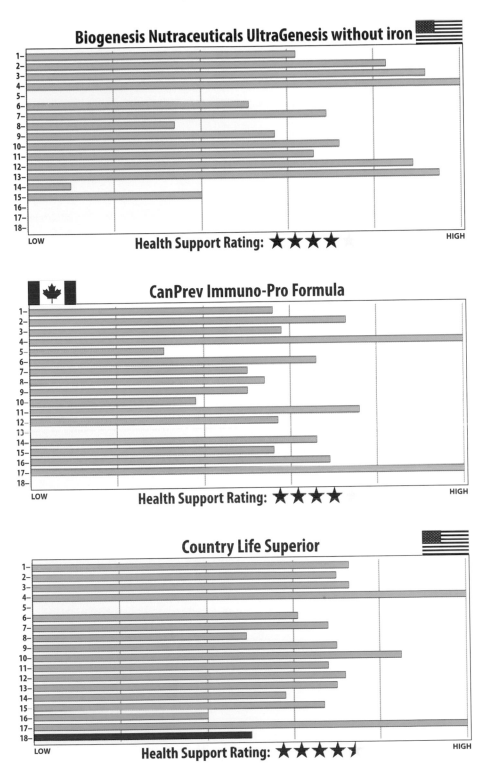

Biogenesis Nutraceuticals UltraGenesis without iron

LOW   **Health Support Rating: ★ ★ ★ ★**   HIGH

CanPrev Immuno-Pro Formula

LOW   **Health Support Rating: ★ ★ ★ ★**   HIGH

Country Life Superior

LOW   **Health Support Rating: ★ ★ ★ ★ ⭒**   HIGH

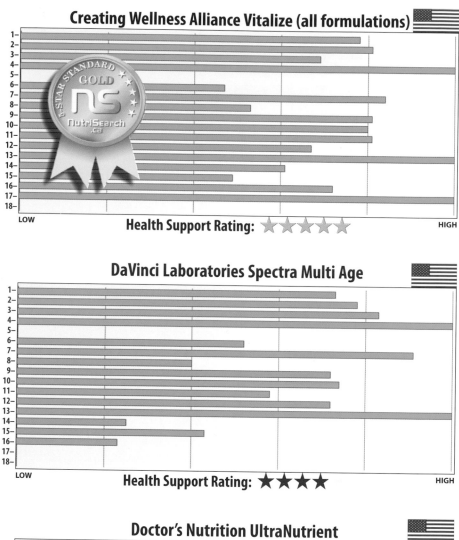

Creating Wellness Alliance Vitalize (all formulations)

Health Support Rating: ★★★★★

LOW   HIGH

DaVinci Laboratories Spectra Multi Age

Health Support Rating: ★★★★

LOW   HIGH

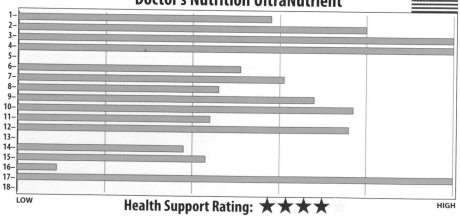

Doctor's Nutrition UltraNutrient

Health Support Rating: ★★★★

LOW   HIGH

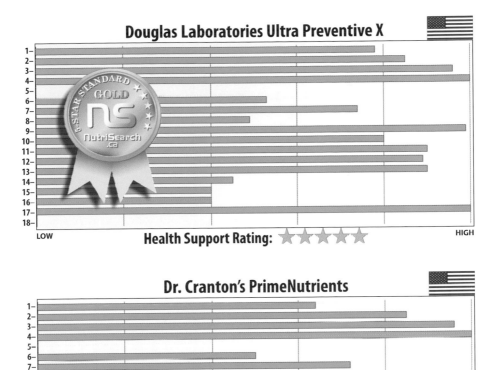

Douglas Laboratories Ultra Preventive X

Health Support Rating: ★★★★★

Dr. Cranton's PrimeNutrients

Health Support Rating: ★★★★

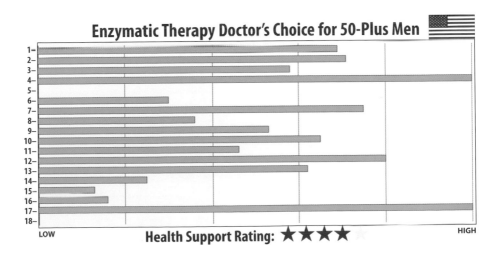

Enzymatic Therapy Doctor's Choice for 50-Plus Men

Health Support Rating: ★★★★

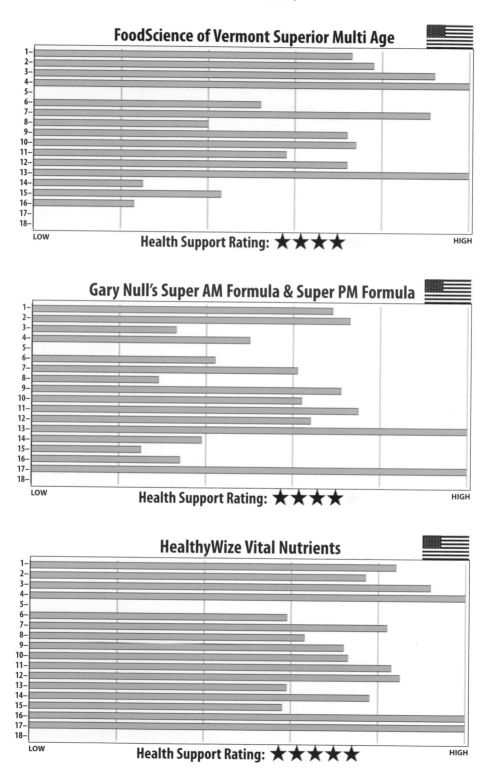

FoodScience of Vermont Superior Multi Age

Health Support Rating: ★★★★

Gary Null's Super AM Formula & Super PM Formula

Health Support Rating: ★★★★

HealthyWize Vital Nutrients

Health Support Rating: ★★★★★

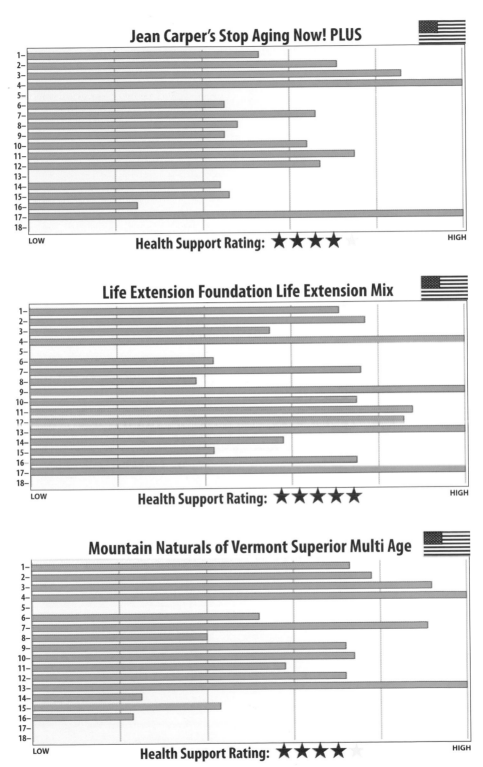

Jean Carper's Stop Aging Now! PLUS

LOW   Health Support Rating: ★★★★   HIGH

Life Extension Foundation Life Extension Mix

LOW   Health Support Rating: ★★★★★   HIGH

Mountain Naturals of Vermont Superior Multi Age

LOW   Health Support Rating: ★★★★   HIGH

SINGLE PRODUCTS, 4-STAR AND HIGHER
(SEE LEGEND ON PAGE 6.2)

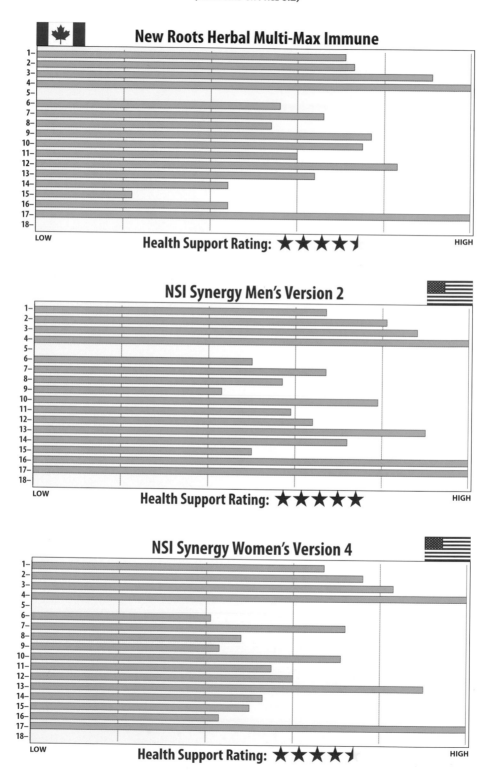

New Roots Herbal Multi-Max Immune

Health Support Rating: ★★★★✦

NSI Synergy Men's Version 2

Health Support Rating: ★★★★★

NSI Synergy Women's Version 4

Health Support Rating: ★★★★✦

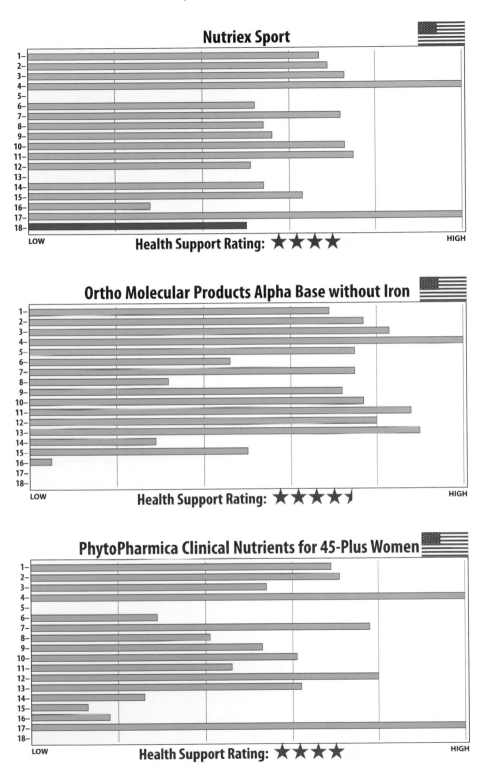

Nutriex Sport

Health Support Rating: ★★★★

Ortho Molecular Products Alpha Base without Iron

Health Support Rating: ★★★★⌐

PhytoPharmica Clinical Nutrients for 45-Plus Women

Health Support Rating: ★★★★

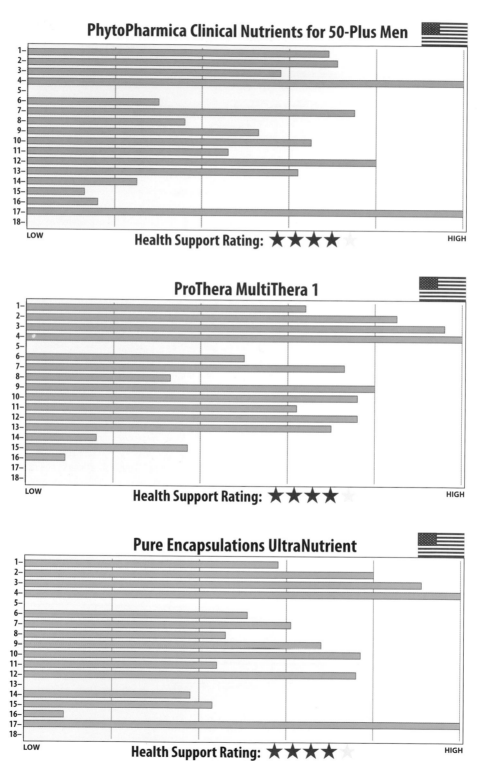

PhytoPharmica Clinical Nutrients for 50-Plus Men

LOW   Health Support Rating: ★★★★☆   HIGH

ProThera MultiThera 1

LOW   Health Support Rating: ★★★★☆   HIGH

Pure Encapsulations UltraNutrient

LOW   Health Support Rating: ★★★★☆   HIGH

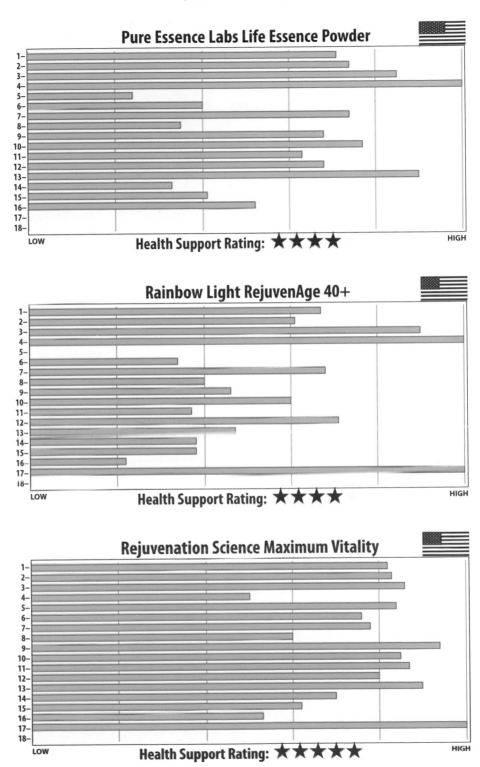

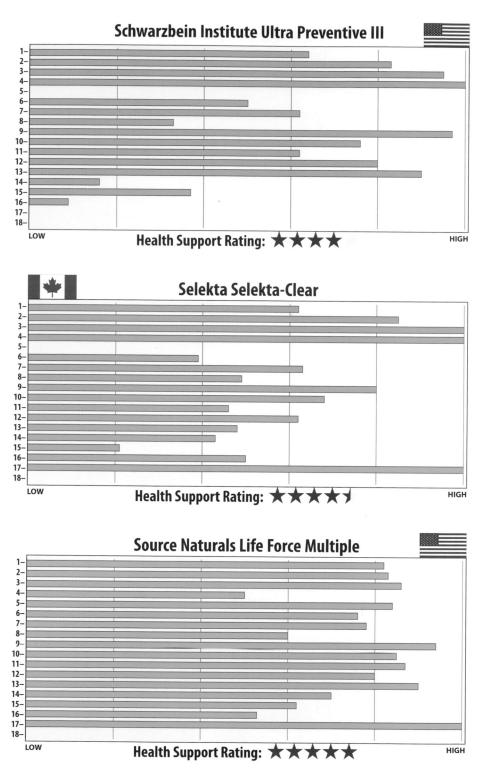

Schwarzbein Institute Ultra Preventive III

Health Support Rating: ★ ★ ★ ★

LOW   HIGH

Selekta Selekta-Clear

Health Support Rating: ★ ★ ★ ★ ⌐

LOW   HIGH

Source Naturals Life Force Multiple

Health Support Rating: ★ ★ ★ ★ ★

LOW   HIGH

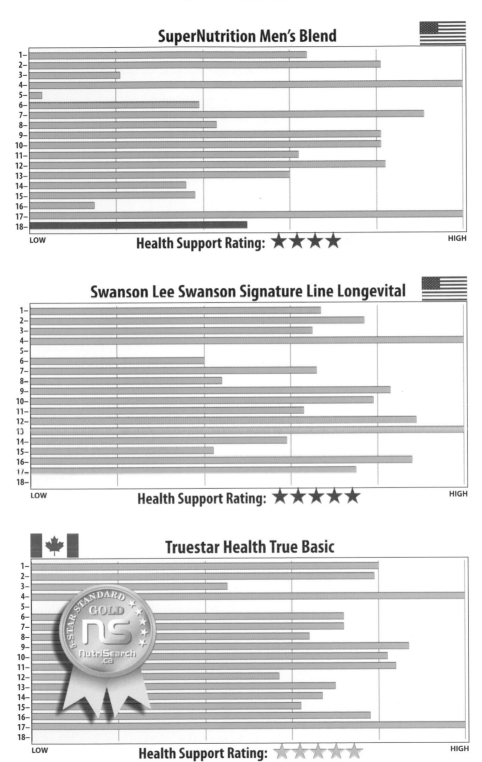

SuperNutrition Men's Blend

LOW   Health Support Rating: ★★★★   HIGH

Swanson Lee Swanson Signature Line Longevital

LOW   Health Support Rating: ★★★★★   HIGH

Truestar Health True Basic

LOW   Health Support Rating: ★★★★★   HIGH

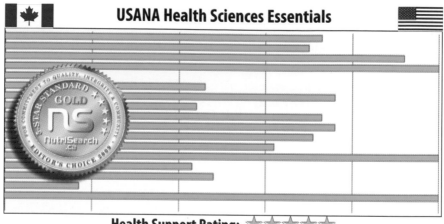

USANA Health Sciences Essentials

Health Support Rating: ★★★★★

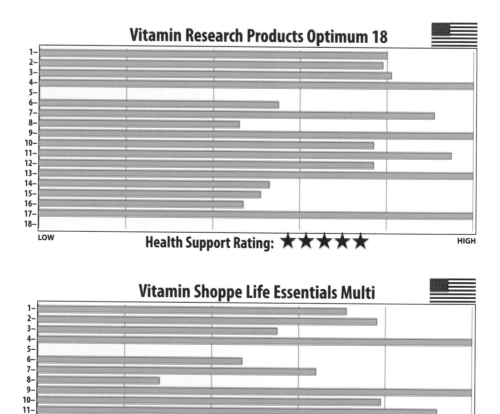

Vitamin Research Products Optimum 18

Health Support Rating: ★★★★★

LOW   HIGH

Vitamin Shoppe Life Essentials Multi

Health Support Rating: ★★★★✦

LOW   HIGH

Health Support Profile Legend

1. Completeness
2. Potency
3. Mineral Forms
4. Bioactivity of Vitamin E
5. Gamma Tocopherol
6. Antioxidant Support
7. Bone Health
8. Heart Health
9. Liver Health

10. Metabolic Health
11. Ocular Health
12. Methylation Support
13. Lipotropic Factors
14. Inflammation Control
15. Glycation Control
16. Bioflavonoid Profile
17. Phenolic Compounds
18. Potential Toxicities

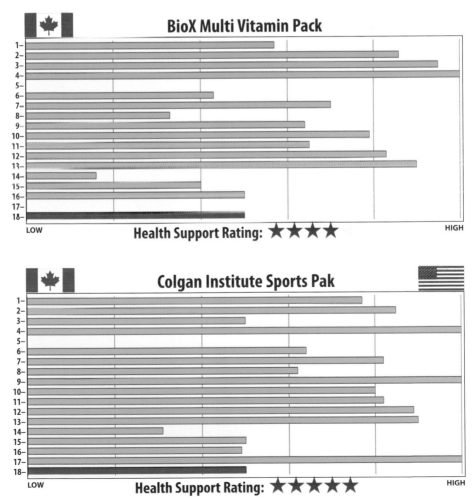

BioX Multi Vitamin Pack

LOW   Health Support Rating: ★★★★   HIGH

Colgan Institute Sports Pak

LOW   Health Support Rating: ★★★★★   HIGH

Douglas Laboratories Daily Core Essentials

1–
2–
3–
4–
5–
6–
7–
8–
9–
10–
11–
12–
13–
14–
15–
16–
17–
18–

LOW   **Health Support Rating:** ★★★★★   HIGH

Douglas Laboratories Longevity Support Pack

1–
2–
3–
4–
5–
6–
7–
8–
9–
10–
11–
12–
13–
14–
15–
16–
17–
18–

LOW   **Health Support Rating:** ★★★★★   HIGH

Jarrow Formulas All Capsule Health Pak

1–
2–
3–
4–
5–
6–
7–
8–
9–
10–
11–
12–
13–
14–
15–
16–
17–
18–

LOW   **Health Support Rating:** ★★★★   HIGH

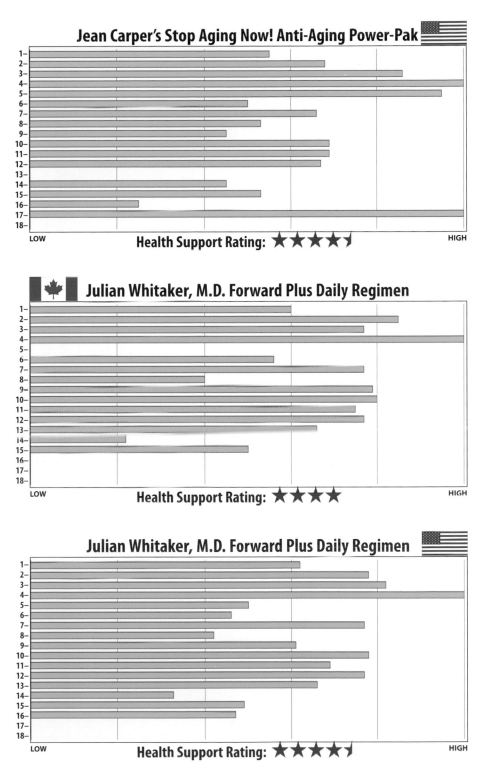

Jean Carper's Stop Aging Now! Anti-Aging Power-Pak

LOW   Health Support Rating: ★★★★⤳   HIGH

Julian Whitaker, M.D. Forward Plus Daily Regimen

LOW   Health Support Rating: ★★★★   HIGH

Julian Whitaker, M.D. Forward Plus Daily Regimen

LOW   Health Support Rating: ★★★★⤳   HIGH

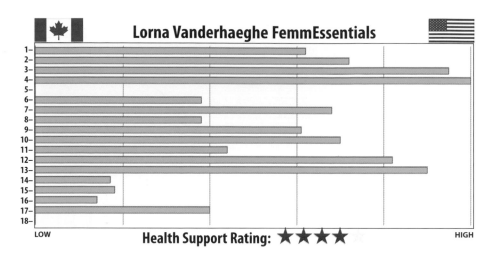

Lorna Vanderhaeghe FemmEssentials

Health Support Rating: ★ ★ ★ ★

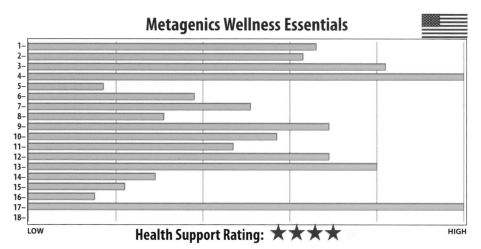

Metagenics Wellness Essentials

Health Support Rating: ★ ★ ★ ★

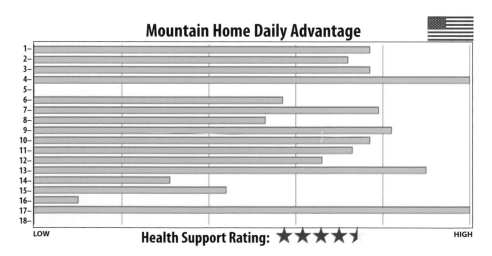

Mountain Home Daily Advantage

Health Support Rating: ★ ★ ★ ★✴

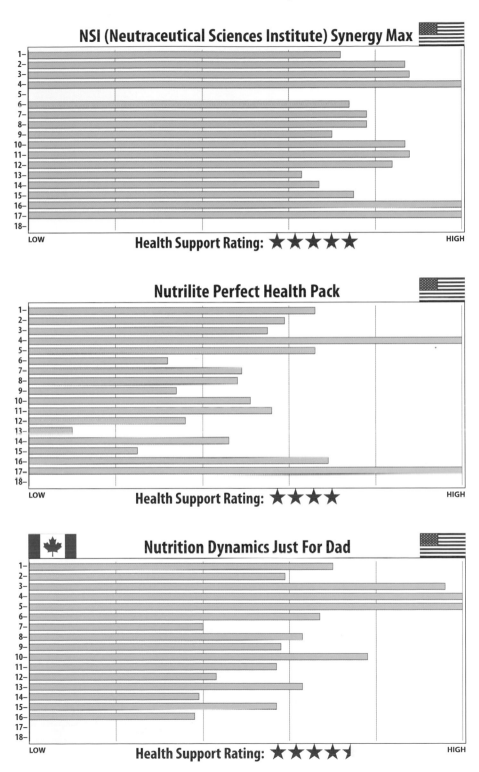

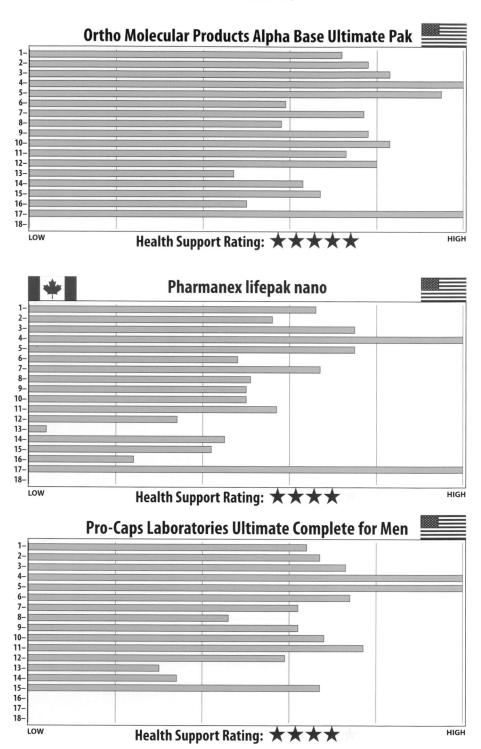

Ortho Molecular Products Alpha Base Ultimate Pak

Health Support Rating: ★ ★ ★ ★ ★

LOW   HIGH

Pharmanex lifepak nano

Health Support Rating: ★ ★ ★ ★

LOW   HIGH

Pro-Caps Laboratories Ultimate Complete for Men

Health Support Rating: ★ ★ ★ ★

LOW   HIGH

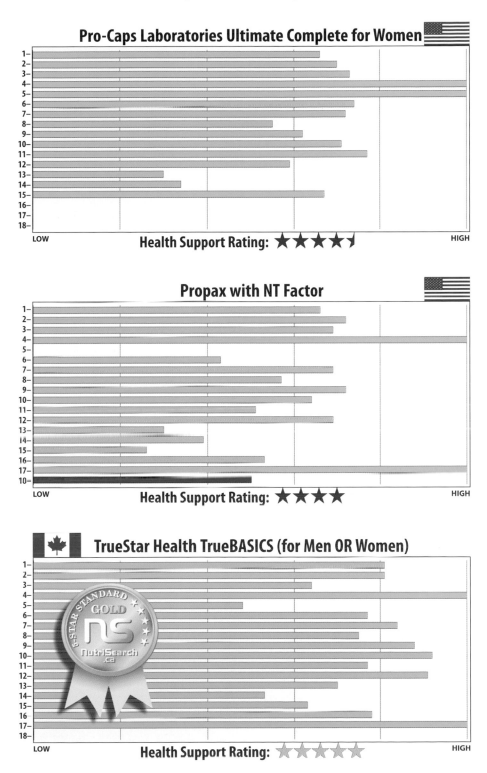

Pro-Caps Laboratories Ultimate Complete for Women

LOW   Health Support Rating: ★ ★ ★ ★ ⁊   HIGH

Propax with NT Factor

LOW   Health Support Rating: ★ ★ ★ ★   HIGH

TrueStar Health TrueBASICS (for Men OR Women)

LOW   Health Support Rating: ★ ★ ★ ★ ★   HIGH

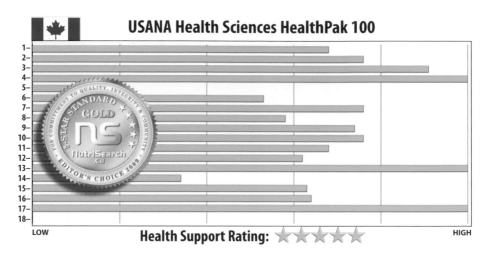

USANA Health Sciences HealthPak 100

LOW   **Health Support Rating:** ★★★★★   HIGH

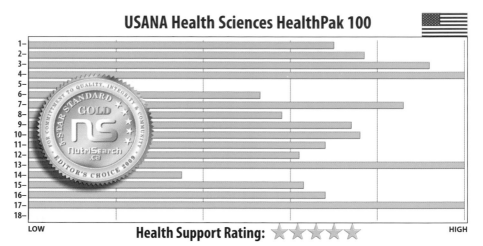

USANA Health Sciences HealthPak 100

LOW   **Health Support Rating:** ★★★★★   HIGH

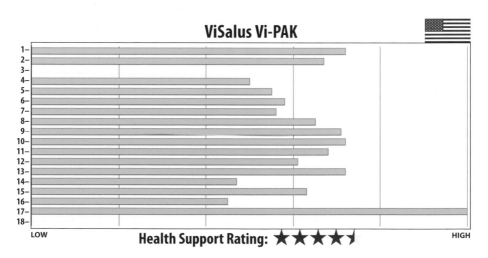

ViSalus Vi-PAK

LOW   **Health Support Rating:** ★★★★✦   HIGH

CHAPTER 7:

SINGLE PRODUCT RATINGS

Sorted Alphabetically by Product Name

SINGLE Product Name	Country	# of Stars
21st Century Mega Multi For Men	US	1½
21st Century Mega Multi For Women	US	2
21st Century One Daily Active	US	½
21st Century One Daily Adults 50+	US	1
21st Century One Daily Carbhealth	US	1
21st Century One Daily Women's	US	0
4Life Multiplex	CA/US	1½
4Life Ritestart Men	US	3
4Life Ritestart Women	US	3
4Life Start Plus	US	2
Action Labs Action Man Multi Once Daily	US	2
Action Labs Action-tabs Made For Men	US	1
Adrien Gagnon Feminex Multi	CA	1
Adrien Gagnon Sélect Multi	CA	1
Advanced Nutritional Innovations (Ani) Coraladvantage	US	1
Advanced Nutritional Innovations (Ani) Coraladvantage Bone & Joint Multi	US	3
Advanced Physician's Products Complete Multivitamin/mineral Without Iron	US	2½
Advanced Physician's Products Maximum Multivitamin/mineral Without Iron	US	3½
Advocare Coreplex	US	2
Agel Min	US	1¼
Agel Min	CA	1½
Alacer Super-gram III	US	1½
Albi Imports Rocky Mountain Multiple	CA	2
Albi Imports Super One A Day	CA	1½
Alive Vitamins Super One Plus	CA	2
All One Multiple For Active Seniors	US	3½
All One Multiple Green Phyto Base	US	3
All One Multiple Original Formula	US	3
All One Multiple Rice Base	US	3
Allergy Research Group Multi-vi-min	US	1½
Allergy Research Group Multi-vi-min Without Copper & Iron	US	2
Allergy Research Group Steady On	US	4
Allergy Research Group Wholly Immune	US	5
Alpha Betic Once-a-day Multi-vitamin	US	1
American Health Nutri Mega	US	2
American Nutrition Ultra Vm-t	US	2
Amni Added Protection III (Copper And Iron Free)	US	3½
Amni Added Protection III (Copper Free With Iron)	US	3½
Amni Added Protection III (Iron Free With Copper)	US	4

SINGLE Product Name	Country	# of Stars
Amni Added Protection III (With Copper & Iron)	US	3½
Amni Basic Preventive 1	US	3½
Amni Basic Preventive 2	US	3½
Amni Basic Preventive 3	US	3½
Amni Basic Preventive 4	US	3½
Amni Basic Preventive 5	US	3½
Amni Basic Preventive 5 Plus Extra Vitamin D	US	4
Amni Essential Basics	US	3
Anabolic Laboratories Aved-digest Multi	US	2
Anabolic Laboratories Aved-multi	US	1½
Anabolic Laboratories Aved-multi Iron Free	US	2
Anabolic Laboratories Multigel Caps	US	2
Aor Essential Mix	CA/US	3
Aor Ortho-core	US	3½
Aor Ortho-core	CA	3
Apex Fitness Fit 50 Plus	US	1
Apex Fitness Fit Performance	US	1
Apex Fitness Fit Vegan/high Carb	US	½
Arbonne Complete Essentials For Men	US	1½
Arbonne Complete Essentials For Women I	US	1
Arbonne Complete Essentials For Women II	US	1
Atkins Basic 3	CA	2
Atkins Basic 3	US	1½
Aumed Coremed	US	2
Avena Originals Vitamin Supreme	CA	2½
Awareness Life Daily Complete	US	1½
Bio-actif Phytobec	CA	½
Biogenesis Nutraceuticals Biofocus	US	1½
Biogenesis Nutraceuticals Ultragenesis	US	3½
Biogenesis Nutraceuticals Ultragenesis Without Iron	US	4
Bio-lumin Essence Daily Essence	US	1½
Biotics Research Corporation Bio-multi Plus	US	1
Biotics Research Corporation Bio-multi Plus Iron & Copper Free	US	1½
Biotics Research Corporation Bio-multi Plus Iron-free	US	1½
Biox Ultimate Once A Day	CA	2½
Bluebonnet Iron Free Multi One	US	2
Bluebonnet Maxi One	US	2
Bluebonnet Maxi Two	US	2½
Bluebonnet Multi One	US	1½
Bluebonnet Multi-vita Softgels	US	2½
Bluebonnet Super Earth Iron-free	US	3
Bluebonnet Super Earth Mini-caplets	US	2½
Bluebonnet Super Earth With Iron	US	2½
Bluebonnet Super Vita-coq10 Formula	US	3½
Body Guard Antioxidant Formula	CA/US	2
Body Rewards Daily Multiple	US	1½
Body Wise Right Choice A.m. + P.m. Formulas	CA/US	3½
Botanic Choice Complete Assurance For Men	US	2
Botanic Choice Complete Assurance For Women	US	2
Botanic Choice High Potency Vitamin & Mineral	US	½

SINGLE Product Name	Country	# of Stars
Botanic Choice Senior Multi-vitamin	US	1½
Botanic Choice Whole Foods Power Multi	US	1½
Bronson Laboratories Fortified Vitamin & Mineral Insurance Formula	US	1½
Bronson Laboratories Mega Multi Softcaps	US	2
Bronson Laboratories Men's Complete Formula With 7-keto	US	2
Bronson Laboratories Multi Formula With Lutein	US	1½
Bronson Laboratories Performance Edge For Men	US	2
Bronson Laboratories Performance Edge For Women	US	2
Bronson Laboratories The Bronson Formula	US	1
Bronson Laboratories Therapeutic Vitamin & Mineral Formula	US	½
Bronson Laboratories Therapeutic Vitamin & Mineral Formula - Without Iron	US	1
Bronson Laboratories Vegi Source	US	3½
Bronson Laboratories Vitamin & Mineral Insurance Formula	US	2
Burns Drugs Multi-max	US	½
Burns Drugs Super-t	US	0
Canadian Sun Formula Flow	CA	1½
Canadian Sun One Plus	CA	2
Canadian Sun Seniors Only	CA	1
Canprev Immuno-pro Formula	CA	4
Carlson Multi-gel	US	2½
Carlson Super 1 Daily	US	1½
Carlson Super 2 Daily	US	2½
Carlson Super-75	US	2
Cell Tech International Alpha Sun	US	0
Cell Tech International Omega Sun	US	0
Centrum	CA	0
Centrum	US	0
Centrum Forte	CA	0
Centrum Advantage	CA	1
Centrum Carb Assist	US	½
Centrum Chewables	US	0
Centrum Liquid	US	0
Centrum Performance	US	½
Centrum Performance	CA	0
Centrum Protegra	CA	½
Centrum Select	CA	½
Centrum Silver	US	½
Centrum Silver Chewables	US	½
Clinician's Formula Vitality Multivite	US	1½
Club Vitamin Best	CA	½
Cnc (Creative Nutrition Canada) Vitamost Plus Formula	CA/US	3
Cnc (Creative Nutrition Canada) Vitamost Prime Formula	CA	2½
Cnc (Creative Nutrition Canada) Vitamost Rtre Formula	CA/US	2½
Colgan Institute First Defense Multi	US	3
Colorado Nutrition Ultimate Men's Formula	US	1½
Colorado Nutrition Ultimate One	US	1
Colorado Nutrition Ultimate Women's Formula	US	1½
Comprehensive Formula Men's	US	1½
Comprehensive Formula Women's	US	1

SINGLE Product Name	Country	# of Stars
COOPER COMPLETE BASIC ONE IRON FREE	US	1
COOPER COMPLETE BASIC ONE WITH IRON	US	1
COOPER COMPLETE IRON FREE	US	2½
COOPER COMPLETE WITH IRON	US	2½
COUNTRY LIFE ADULT MULTI	US	1
COUNTRY LIFE BEYOND FOOD	US	3
COUNTRY LIFE DAILY TOTAL ONE	US	1½
COUNTRY LIFE ENHANCED QM-1	US	1½
COUNTRY LIFE ESSSENTIAL LIFE	US	2½
COUNTRY LIFE GREEN EDGE II	US	1½
COUNTRY LIFE MAX FOR MEN	US	3
COUNTRY LIFE MAXINE FOR WOMEN	US	2½
COUNTRY LIFE MAXINE FOR WOMEN IRON-FREE	US	3
COUNTRY LIFE MAXINE FOR WOMEN VEGETARIAN CAPS	US	2½
COUNTRY LIFE MULTI-100	US	2
COUNTRY LIFE SENIORITY	US	1½
COUNTRY LIFE SUPERIOR	US	4½
COUNTRY LIFE VEGETARIAN SUPPORT	US	2
CREATING WELLNESS ALLIANCE VITALIZE MEN'S FORMULA	US	5 GOLD
CREATING WELLNESS ALLIANCE VITALIZE WOMEN'S FORMULA	US	5 GOLD
CREATING WELLNESS ALLIANCE VITALIZE SENIOR WOMEN'S GOLD FORMULA	US	5 GOLD
CURVES COMPLETE	US	1½
CURVES COMPLETE BIOMULTIPLE	US	1½
CURVES MULTIVITAMIN	CA	2
CURVES PROTEIN DRINK	US	0
CVS PHARMACY DAILY MULTIPLE 50 PLUS	US	½
CVS PHARMACY DAILY MULTIPLE FOR MEN	US	½
CVS PHARMACY DAILY MULTIPLE FOR WOMEN	US	0
CVS PHARMACY MEGA MULTI	US	2
CVS PHARMACY MULTIVITAMIN & MINERALS	US	0
CVS PHARMACY SPECTRAVITE	US	0
CVS PHARMACY SPECTRAVITE PERFORMANCE	US	½
CVS PHARMACY SPECTRAVITE SENIOR	US	½
CVS PHARMACY SPECTRAVITE SENIOR CHEWABLES	US	½
CVS PHARMACY THERA PLUS	US	½
CVS PHARMACY TODAY'S LIFE MEN'S	US	1
CVS PHARMACY TODAY'S LIFE WOMEN'S	US	1½
CVS PHARMACY TODAY'S LIFE 50+	US	½
CVS PHARMACY TODAY'S LIFE ACTIVE+	US	½
CVS PHARMACY WEIGHT SHARP	US	1
CYTO CHARGE LIFE ASSURANCE	US	2½
DAVINCI LABORATORIES DAILY BEST	US	2
DAVINCI LABORATORIES GENESSENTIALS SPECTRA SNP	US	3½
DAVINCI LABORATORIES OMNI	US	1½
DAVINCI LABORATORIES SPECTRA	US	3½
DAVINCI LABORATORIES SPECTRA MAN	US	3½
DAVINCI LABORATORIES SPECTRA MULTI AGE	US	4
DAVINCI LABORATORIES SPECTRA SENIOR	US	3½
DAVINCI LABORATORIES SPECTRA WITHOUT COPPER & IRON	US	3½
DAVINCI LABORATORIES SPECTRA WOMAN	US	3½

SINGLE Product Name	Country	# of Stars
Dc (Dee Cee Laboratories) 6bg+	US	½
Dc (Dee Cee Laboratories) Formula 19	US	½
Dc (Dee Cee Laboratories) Formula 249 Iron Free	US	1
Dc (Dee Cee Laboratories) Formula 360	US	½
Dc (Dee Cee Laboratories) Formula 75	US	1½
Dc (Dee Cee Laboratories) Formula 784	US	0
Dc (Dee Cee Laboratories) Formula 814	US	½
Dc (Dee Cee Laboratories) Ultra Vm	US	1½
Dc (Dee Cee Laboratories) Vidoplex-ml	US	½
Designs For Health Dfh Complete Multi	US	3
Designs For Health Dfh Complete Multi Without Copper & Iron	US	3
Doctor's Nutrition Mega Vites Man	US	3½
Doctor's Nutrition Mega Vites Senior	US	3
Doctor's Nutrition Mega Vites Without Copper & Iron	US	3½
Doctor's Nutrition Mega Vites Woman	US	3½
Doctor's Nutrition Ultranutrient	US	4
Don Lemmon's All Natural Balanced Multi-nutrient	US	3½
Douglas Laboratories Added Protection III	US	3½
Douglas Laboratories Added Protection III Copper & Iron Free	US	3½
Douglas Laboratories Added Protection III Copper Free	US	3½
Douglas Laboratories Added Protection III Iron Free	US	4
Douglas Laboratories Basic Preventive 1	US	3½
Douglas Laboratories Basic Preventive 2	US	3½
Douglas Laboratories Basic Preventive 3	US	3½
Douglas Laboratories Basic Preventive 4	US	3½
Douglas Laboratories Basic Preventive 5	US	3½
Douglas Laboratories Basic Preventive 5 Plus Extra Vitamin D	US	4
Douglas Laboratories Essential Basics	US	3
Douglas Laboratories Geri-vite 25	US	1
Douglas Laboratories Multivite	US	0
Douglas Laboratories Nutri-smart Formula	US	2½
Douglas Laboratories Ultra Balance III (Capsules)	CA	2½
Douglas Laboratories Ultra Balance III (Tablets)	CA	4
Douglas Laboratories Ultra Balance III With Iron (Tablets)	CA	3½
Douglas Laboratories Ultra Fem	US	3
Douglas Laboratories Ultra Preventive Beta	US	3½
Douglas Laboratories Ultra Preventive Beta With Copper	US	3½
Douglas Laboratories Ultra Preventive Beta With Copper & Iron	US	3½
Douglas Laboratories Ultra Preventive D	US	3½
Douglas Laboratories Ultra Preventive D With Copper	US	4
Douglas Laboratories Ultra Preventive D With Copper & Iron	US	3½
Douglas Laboratories Ultra Preventive III (Capsules)	US	3
Douglas Laboratories Ultra Preventive III (Tablets)	US	4
Douglas Laboratories Ultra Preventive III With Copper & Iron (Tablets)	US	3½
Douglas Laboratories Ultra Preventive III With Copper (Capsules)	US	2½
Douglas Laboratories Ultra Preventive III With Copper (Tablets)	US	4
Douglas Laboratories Ultra Preventive III With Iron (Tablets)	US	3
Douglas Laboratories Ultra Preventive III With Zinc Picolinate (Tablets)	US	3

SINGLE Product Name	Country	# of Stars
DOUGLAS LABORATORIES ULTRA PREVENTIVE IX	US	5 GOLD
DOUGLAS LABORATORIES ULTRA PREVENTIVE IX WITH VITAMIN K	US	5 GOLD
DOUGLAS LABORATORIES ULTRA PREVENTIVE X	CA/US	5 GOLD
DOUGLAS LABORATORIES ULTRA VITE 75 II	US	1
DOUGLAS LABORATORIES ULTRA-AM & ULTRA-PM	US	4
DOUGLAS LABORATORIES VITA-CHEL-PLUS	US	2½
DOUGLAS LABORATORIES VITAWORX	US	3½
DR. CRANTON'S PRIMENUTRIENTS	US	4
DR. DONSBACH'S ORA-FLO	US	2½
DR. FUHRMAN'S GENTLE CARE FORMULA	US	1
DR. RATH'S VITACOR PLUS	US	1
DR. RATH'S WOMEN'S HEALTH PROGRAM	US	2
DRINKABLES MULTI VITAMINS FOR SENIORS	US	½
DRUCKER LABS INTRAMAX	US	2½
ECLECTIC INSTITUTE OPTI GYN FORMULA	CA/US	3½
ECLECTIC INSTITUTE VITAL FORCE	US	3
ECONUGENICS MEN'S LONGEVITY ESSENTIALS PLUS	US	1½
ECONUGENICS WOMEN'S LONGEVITY RHYTHMS	US	2
ECONUGENICS WOMEN'S LONGEVITY RHYTHMS GOLD	US	2
ENDURANCE PRODUCTS ENDUR-VM	US	½
ENDURANCE PRODUCTS ENDUR-VM WITHOUT IRON	US	½
ENEREX SONA	CA	2
ENEREX SONA RX	CA	2½
ENIVA ESSENTIAL PHYTAMINS & CELL-READY MINERALS (CRANBERRY-GRAPEFRUIT BLEND)	US	1½
ENIVA ESSENTIAL PHYTAMINS AND CELL-READY MINERALS (ORIGINAL FORMULA)	US	1½
ENIVA VIBE	US	1½
ENZYMATIC THERAPY DOCTOR'S CHOICE FOR 45-PLUS WOMEN	US	3½
ENZYMATIC THERAPY DOCTOR'S CHOICE FOR 50-PLUS MEN	US	4
ENZYMATIC THERAPY DOCTOR'S CHOICE FOR MEN	CA	3½
ENZYMATIC THERAPY DOCTOR'S CHOICE FOR MEN	US	3½
ENZYMATIC THERAPY DOCTOR'S CHOICE FOR WOMEN	US	3½
ENZYME LABS NUTRACEUTICALS MULTI-LIFE	US	1½
EPIC4HEALTH PHYSICIAN'S MULTI VITAMIN FORMULA	US	2
EQUALINE CENTRAL-VITE	US	0
EQUALINE CENTRAL-VITE CARB DIETER FORMULA	US	½
EQUALINE CENTRAL-VITE PERFORMANCE	US	½
EQUALINE CENTRAL-VITE SELECT	US	½
EQUALINE ONE DAILY 50 PLUS	US	½
EQUALINE ONE DAILY ACTIVE	US	½
EQUALINE ONE DAILY DIETER'S SUPPORT FORMULA	US	1
EQUALINE ONE DAILY MAXIMUM	US	0
EQUALINE ONE DAILY MEN'S HEALTH FORMULA	US	½
EQUALINE ONE DAILY WOMEN'S	US	0
EQUATE CENTURY COMPLETE	CA	0
EQUATE CENTURY PERFORM	CA	0
EQUATE CENTURY PLUS	CA	0
EQUATE CENTURY PREMIUM	CA	½
EQUATE CENTURY SILVER	CA	½

SINGLE Product Name	Country	# of Stars
EQUATE CENTURY SILVER CHEWABLE	CA	½
EQUATE COMPLETE	US	0
EQUATE COMPLETE MATURE	US	½
EQUATE ONE DAILY MEN'S	CA	½
EQUATE ONE DAILY MEN'S	US	½
EQUATE ONE DAILY WOMEN'S	US	0
EQUATE ONE TABLET DAILY	CA	½
EQUATE ONE TABLET DAILY ADULTS	CA	0
EQUATE ONE TABLET DAILY ADULTS 50+	CA	½
EQUATE ONE TABLET DAILY WOMEN'S	CA	0
ESSENCE-OF-LIFE LIQUID NUTRITION PLUS/ESSENCE	US	2
ESSENCE-OF-LIFE ONLY ONE CELL-READY NUTRITION	US	1
EXACT ESSENTRA BALANCE	CA	0
EXACT ESSENTRA ELITE	CA	½
EXACT ESSENTRA FORTE	CA	0
EXACT ESSENTRA PLATINUM	CA	½
EXACT FOR ADULTS OVER 50	CA	0
EXACT MULTI MAX 1	CA	2
EXACT VITAL ONE MEN'S FORMULA	CA	½
EXACT VITAL-FEM 1	CA	0
FIRST ORGANICS DAILY MULTIPLE	US	1
FLORA MULTI VITAMINS	CA	2
FOODSCIENCE OF VERMONT DAILY BEST	US	2
FOODSCIENCE OF VERMONT MEN'S SUPERIOR	US	3½
FOODSCIENCE OF VERMONT SENIOR'S SUPERIOR	US	3½
FOODSCIENCE OF VERMONT SUPERIOR CARE	US	3
FOODSCIENCE OF VERMONT SUPERIOR CARE WITHOUT COPPER AND IRON	US	3½
FOODSCIENCE OF VERMONT SUPERIOR MULTI AGE	US	4
FOODSCIENCE OF VERMONT TOTAL CARE	US	1½
FOODSCIENCE OF VERMONT WOMEN'S SUPERIOR	US	3½
FORMOR INTERNATIONAL ANOX	US	2
FREEDA MONOCAPS	US	½
FREEDA QUINTABS-M	US	1
FREEDA QUINTABS-M IRON-FREE	US	1½
FREEDA ULTRA FREEDA, A-FREE	US	2
FREEDA ULTRA FREEDA, IRON-FREE	US	2½
FREEDA ULTRA FREEDA, WITH IRON	US	2½
FUTURE FORMULATIONS ADVANCE (IRON FREE)	CA	1½
FUTUREBIOTICS HI ENERGY MULTI FOR MEN	US	2
FUTUREBIOTICS MULTIVITAMIN ENERGY PLUS FOR WOMEN	US	1½
FUTUREBIOTICS VEGETARIAN SUPER MULTI	US	2
GARDEN OF LIFE LIVING MULTI	CA	1½
GARDEN OF LIFE LIVING MULTI	US	2
GARDEN OF LIFE LIVING MULTI IRON FREE	CA	2
GARDEN OF LIFE LIVING MULTI MEN'S FORMULA	CA/US	2
GARDEN OF LIFE LIVING MULTI OPTIMAL WOMEN'S FORMULA	CA	1½
GARDEN OF LIFE LIVING MULTI OPTIMAL WOMEN'S FORMULA	US	1½
GARY NULL'S SUPER AM FORMULA	US	2
GARY NULL'S SUPER AM FORMULA & SUPER PM FORMULA	US	4
GARY NULL'S SUPER PM FORMULA	US	1½

SINGLE Product Name	Country	# of Stars
GENESIS TODAY 4 TOTAL NUTRITION	US	3
GENUINE HEALTH GREENS+ MULTI+	CA	3
GENUINE HEALTH GREENS+ MULTI+ POWDER	CA	3½
GENUINE HEALTH GREENS+ MULTI+ TABLETS	CA	2½
GENUINE HEALTH MULTI+ COMPLETE	CA	3
GENUINE HEALTH MULTI+ DAILY TRIM	CA	2
GERITOL COMPLETE	US	0
GLOBAL HEALTH TRAX (GHT) DAILY VITA PLUS & MEGA MINERALS PLUS	US	2
GNC CHEWABLE SOLOTRON	US	½
GNC MEGA MEN	CA	1½
GNC MEGA MEN	US	2½
GNC MEGA MEN 50 PLUS	US	2
GNC MULTI LIQUID ULTRA MEGA	US	3
GNC MULTI PREVENTRON	US	1
GNC MULTI SOLOTRON	CA	1
GNC MULTI SOLOTRON	US	1
GNC MULTI SOLOTRON PLATINUM	US	1
GNC MULTI SOLOTRON WITHOUT IRON	US	1½
GNC MULTI ULTRA MEGA	CA	1½
GNC MULTI ULTRA MEGA	US	1½
GNC MULTI ULTRA MEGA GOLD	US	2½
GNC MULTI ULTRA MEGA GOLD WITHOUT IRON	US	2½
GNC MULTI ULTRA MEGA GREEN	US	2
GNC MULTI ULTRA MEGA SOFTGELS	CA	2
GNC MULTI-GEL	US	1½
GNC PLATINUM YEARS	CA	1
GNC PREVENTIVE NUTRITION MEN'S MULTIPLE	US	1½
GNC PREVENTIVE NUTRITION PREMIUM ONE WITHOUT IRON	US	1½
GNC PREVENTIVE NUTRITION WOMEN'S MULTIPLE	US	1½
GNC WOMEN'S ULTRA MEGA	CA	2
GNC WOMEN'S ULTRA MEGA WITHOUT IRON	CA	2
GNC WOMEN'S WOMEN'S ULTRA MEGA	US	2
GNC WOMEN'S WOMEN'S ULTRA MEGA BONE DENSITY	US	2
GNLD INTERNATIONAL FORMULA IV	US	1
GNLD INTERNATIONAL FORMULA IV PLUS	US	1½
GNLD INTERNATIONAL VEGETARIAN MULTI	US	1
GOLDSHIELD CENTURAL SILVER	US	½
GOLDSHIELD TOTAL MULTIVITAMIN & MINERAL FORMULA	US	2
GOOD NEIGHBOR PHARMACY CENTURY	US	0
GOOD NEIGHBOR PHARMACY CENTURY ADVANTAGE	US	½
GOOD NEIGHBOR PHARMACY CENTURY SENIOR	US	½
GOOD NEIGHBOR PHARMACY MAXIMUM ONE DAILY	US	½
GOOD NEIGHBOR PHARMACY ONE DAILY CARB-VANTAGE	US	½
GOOD NEIGHBOR PHARMACY THERAPEUTIC-M COMPLETE	US	½
GOOD NEIGHBOR PHARMACY WOMEN'S ONE DAILY	US	0
GREAT AMERICAN PRODUCTS MASTER GREEN MULTI	US	2½
GREAT EARTH SUPER HY-VITES EXTRA STRENGTH	US	2
GREAT EARTH SUPER HY-VITES REGULAR STRENGTH	US	1½
GREAT EARTH SUPER HY-VITES ULTRA STRENGTH	US	2½
GREAT EARTH TNT EXTRA STRENGTH TIMED RELEASE	US	3½

SINGLE Product Name	Country	# of Stars
Greens+ Greens+ Powder	US	1½
Health First Iron Free Multi-first	CA	2
Health First Multi-first	CA	1½
Healthywize Vital Greens	US	4½
Healthywize Vital Nutrients	US	5
Heaven Sent Naturals Balanced Essentials	US	1
H-e-b Complete	US	0
H-e-b Complete Advantage	US	½
H-e-b Complete Senior	US	½
H-e-b Multiple Vitamins Men's	US	½
H-e-b Multiple Vitamins 50 Plus	US	½
H-e-b Multiple Vitamins Maximum	US	0
H-e-b Therapeutic-m	US	½
Henry's Farmer's Market 75 Complete	US	2
Henry's Farmer's Market Basic Multi	US	½
Henry's Farmer's Market Iron Free Basic Multi	US	½
Henry's Farmer's Market Iron Free Multi Caps	US	2
Henry's Farmer's Market Iron Free Ultimate One	US	2
Henry's Farmer's Market Life Multi Complete	US	2
Henry's Farmer's Market Softgel Multi	US	2
Henry's Farmer's Market Ultimate Capsule	US	1½
Henry's Farmer's Market Ultimate One	US	2
Henry's Farmer's Market Ultimate Two	US	2
Henry's Farmer's Market Ultimate Vegetarian Multi	US	2
Henry's Marketplace Ultimate Senior Multi	US	1½
Herbalife Shapeworks Garden 7	US	1
Herbalife Shapeworks Multivitamin Complex (Formula 2)	US	1
Herbasway Laboratories Multivitamin Magic & Multimineral Magic	US	1½
Highland Laboratories Energy With Whole Food Concentrates	US	3
Highland Laboratories Mega I Daily	US	1½
Highland Laboratories Mega I Daily Iron-free	US	1½
Highland Laboratories Mega II Daily	US	2
Highland Laboratories Mega II Daily Iron-free	US	2
Highland Laboratories Men's 30 Plus Multi	US	2½
Highland Laboratories Nature's Daily	US	1
Highland Laboratories Omni	US	2½
Highland Laboratories Women's 30 Plus Multi	US	2½
Hillestad Pharmaceuticals Sterling	US	2
Hillestad Pharmaceuticals Summit Gold	US	1½
Hillestad Pharmaceuticals Summit Gold Special Formula	US	2
Hillestad Pharmaceuticals Vitamin/mineral Complex Unit A	US	1
Holista Advanz	US	1½
Holista Advanz Iron Free	US	1½
Immunotec Research Vitamin/mineral Supplement	CA	½
Immuvit Original Swiss Formula	US	½
Innate Response Formulas Biomax Food Multi III	US	½
Innate Response Formulas Food Multi II	US	1
Innate Response Formulas Food Multi IV	US	2½
Innate Response Formulas Men Over 40	US	2½
Innate Response Formulas Men's Multi	US	1

SINGLE Product Name	Country	# of Stars
Innate Response Formulas Men's Multi Without Iron	US	1½
Innate Response Formulas Men's One Daily	US	½
Innate Response Formulas One Daily I	US	½
Innate Response Formulas One Daily II	US	½
Innate Response Formulas Women Over 40	US	2
Innate Response Formulas Women's Multi	US	1
Innate Response Formulas Women's One Daily	US	½
Inno-vite Formula H.H.	CA	1½
Inno-vite Total Nrg Lift	CA	1½
Intelligent Nutrients Nutribase	US	2
Intensive Nutrition Mega-vm	US	2½
Intensive Nutrition Multi-vm	US	3
Isagenix Essentials For Men	CA	1½
Isagenix Essentials For Men	US	1½
Isagenix Essentials For Women	US	1½
Isagenix Women's Essentials	CA	1½
Isotonix Champion Blend	US	2
Isotonix Multitech	US	1
Isotonix Multitech With Iron	US	½
Jamieson Power Vitamins For Men	CA	1½
Jamieson Regular Vita-vim	CA	1
Jamieson Stamina	CA	½
Jamieson Super Vita-vim	CA	1½
Jamieson Vita Slim	CA	1½
Jamieson Vita-vim Adult 50+	CA	1
Jamieson Vita-vim Adult Chewable	CA	½
Jarrow Formulas Longevity Multi	US	3½
Jarrow Formulas Multi 1-to-3	US	2½
Jarrow Formulas Multi Easy Powder	CA/US	2½
Jarrow Formulas Women's Multi	CA/US	2
Jean Carper's Stop Aging Now!	US	4
Jean Carper's Stop Aging Now! Plus	US	4
Julian Whitaker, M.D. Forward Multi-nutrient	US	3
Juvio Rejuvionate Green Perfection	CA/US	1½
Kal Enhanced Energy	US	3
Kal Enhanced-75	US	2
Kal High Potency Soft Multiple Iron Free	US	2
Kal Mega Vita-min	US	2
Kal Multi-active	US	3
Kal Multi-four+	US	2½
Kal Multi-max 1	US	2
Kal Multiple Energy	US	2½
Kal Softone Multi With Lutein	US	1½
Kal Vitality For Women	US	2
Karuna Him	US	3
Karuna Maxxum 1	US	3
Karuna Maxxum 2	US	3
Karuna Maxxum 3	US	3
Karuna Maxxum 4	US	3½
Kirkland Daily Multi	US	½

SINGLE Product Name	Country	# of Stars
KIRKLAND FORMULA FORTE	CA	0
KIRKLAND PREMIUM PERFORMANCE MULTIVITAMIN	US	½
KIRKMAN EVERYDAY	US	½
KIRKMAN EVERYDAY & NUTHERA EVERYDAY COMPANION CAPSULES	US	1½
KIRKMAN NU-THERA WITHOUT VITAMINS A & D	US	1
KIRKMAN SUPER NU-THERA	US	1
KLAMATH BLUE GREEN ALGAE	US	½
KLAMATH POWER 3	US	½
KROGER COMPLETE	US	0
KROGER FORTIFY	US	½
KROGER MEN	US	1½
KROGER ONE DAILY MAXIMUM	US	0
KROGER ONE DAILY MEN'S HEALTH FORMULA	US	½
KROGER ONE DAILY WOMEN'S HEALTH	US	0
KROGER THERA PLUS	US	½
LA WEIGHT LOSS CENTERS VITA-MAX	CA	1
LEADER CENTURY	US	0
LEADER CENTURY SENIOR	US	½
LEADER MEN'S ONE DAILY	US	½
LEADER WOMEN'S ONE DAILY	US	0
LEVITY+PLUS MULTIVITAMIN FOR WOMEN	US	2
LIFE ADULT	CA	0
LIFE CHEWABLE TABLETS	CA	½
LIFE DAILY-ONE 50+	CA	½
LIFE DAILY-ONE ADULT	CA	0
LIFE DAILY-ONE CARB SENSE	CA	½
LIFE DAILY-ONE FOR WOMEN	CA	0
LIFE DAILY-ONE MEN'S FORMULA	CA	½
LIFE DAILY-ONE WEIGHT SENSE	CA	1
LIFE EXTENSION FOUNDATION LIFE EXTENSION MIX	US	5
LIFE FOR PEOPLE OVER 50	CA	0
LIFE OPTIMUM	CA	½
LIFE OPTIMUM 50+	CA	½
LIFE PLUS DAILY BIOBASICS	US	2½
LIFE SOLUTIONS SUPER MULTI VITAMINS AND MINERALS	US	2½
LIFE SPECTRUM	CA	0
LIFE SPECTRUM GOLD	CA	½
LIFE SPECTRUM PERFORMA	CA	½
LIFE SPECTRUM WITH BETA CAROTENE	CA	1½
LIFE-LINE DAILY PLUS 50	US	½
LIFE-LINE MAXIMUM DAILY GREENS	US	2
LIFE-LINE THERAVITS 100	US	2½
LIFESCRIPT DAILY ESSENTIALS, PLUS CALCIUM COMPLETE	US	1
LIFESOURCE NUTRITION LIQUID MULTI VITAMIN & IMMUNE BOOSTER	US	1½
LIFESOURCE NUTRITION MULTI VITAMIN & MINERALS	US	2½
LIFESTYLES LIFECYCLES FOR MATURE MEN	CA/US	1
LIFESTYLES LIFECYCLES FOR MATURE WOMEN	CA/US	1
LIFESTYLES LIFECYCLES FOR MEN	CA/US	1
LIFESTYLES LIFECYCLES FOR WOMEN	CA/US	1
LIFETIME ADULT VIT-MINS	US	1

SINGLE Product Name	Country	# of Stars
LIFETIME LIFE'S BASICS	US	2
LIFETIME MULTI-VITAMIN & MINERAL SOFT GELS	US	2
LIFETIME NUTRILIFE SOFT GELS	CA	1
LIQUID HEALTH DAILY MULTIPLE	US	½
LIQUIMAX COMPLETE NUTRITION	US	1
LONDON DRUGS MULTI COMPLETE	CA	0
LONDON DRUGS MULTI PLUS	CA	½
LONDON DRUGS MULTI PREMIUM	CA	1
LONDON DRUGS MULTI SILVER	CA	1
LONDON DRUGS MULTI VITAMIN & MINERALS	CA	½
LONDON DRUGS ONE ADULTS 50+	CA	1
LONDON DRUGS ONE TABLET DAILY ADULTS	CA	½
LONDON DRUGS WOMEN'S FORMULA	CA	0
LONDON NATURALS IRON-FREE	CA	2
LONDON NATURALS PREMIER	CA	2
LONGEVITY SCIENCE REVITALIZE	US	3
LONGS ADVANCED FORMULA CENTRAL VITE	US	0
LONGS CENTRAL VITE CARB DIETER FORMULA	US	½
LONGS CENTRAL VITE PERFORMANCE	US	½
LONGS CENTRAL VITE SELECT	US	½
LONGS MEN'S MULTIVITAMIN/MINERAL SUPPLEMENT WITH HERBS	US	2
LONGS ONE DAILY DIETER'S SUPPORT FORMULA	US	1
LONGS ONE DAILY MEN'S HEALTH FORMULA	US	½
LONGS ONE DAILY WOMEN'S	US	0
LONGS THERA PLUS	US	0
LONGS WELLNESS HIGH POTENCY MULTI VITAMIN & MINERAL	US	0
LONGS WOMEN'S MULTIVITAMIN/MULTIMINERAL/HERBS	US	1
MAJESTIC EARTH ULTIMATE CLASSIC	US	3
MAJESTIC EARTH ULTIMATE DAILY	US	1½
MANNATECH GLYCENTIALS	US	2½
MANNATECH GLYCENTIALS	CA	2
MASON DAILY MULTIPLE VITAMINS WITH MINERALS	US	0
MASON SUPER MULTIPLE	US	1
MASON VITATRUM COMPLETE	US	0
MASON VITATRUM ENDURANCE	US	½
MASON VITRUM SENIOR	US	½
MATOL MEGAVITAMINS	CA	2
MATOL MEGAVITAMINS	US	2
MAXION FORMULA F-L-W	CA	1½
MAXION NUTRITION ARTR-E-CLNZ	US	1½
MAXION NUTRITION MAX MULTI LIQUID VITAMIN	CA/US	1
MAXIVISION WHOLE BODY FORMULA	US	3
MD HEALTHLINE AD-DITIONS	US	1
MD HEALTHLINE ADVANCED GREEN MULTI FORMULA	US	0
MD'S CHOICE COMPLETE FORMULA FOR MATURE WOMEN	US	3
MD'S CHOICE COMPLETE FORMULA FOR MEN	US	3
MD'S CHOICE COMPLETE FORMULA FOR YOUNG WOMEN	US	3
MEGAFOOD ALPHA DAILYFOODS	US	1½
MEGAFOOD ESSENTIALS FOODBASED MINI'S	US	2½
MEGAFOOD ESSENTIALS FOR MENOPAUSE	US	2½

SINGLE PRODUCT NAME	COUNTRY	# OF STARS
MEGAFOOD ESSENTIALS IRON FREE ONE DAILY	US	1½
MEGAFOOD ESSENTIALS ONE DAILY	US	1½
MEGAFOOD IRON FREE ONE DAILY	US	½
MEGAFOOD LIFESTYLE DAILYFOODS	US	2
MEGAFOOD MAXIMUM LIFE	US	3
MEGAFOOD MAXIMUM MAN	US	2
MEGAFOOD MAXIMUM MAN ONE DAILY	US	1
MEGAFOOD MAXIMUM WOMAN	US	2
MEGAFOOD MAXIMUM WOMAN ONE DAILY	US	1
MEGAFOOD MEDI-SAFE DAILYFOODS	US	½
MEGAFOOD MEN OVER 40 DAILYFOODS	US	2
MEGAFOOD MEN'S DAILYFOODS	US	½
MEGAFOOD MEN'S ONE DAILY DAILYFOODS	US	0
MEGAFOOD ONE DAILY DAILYFOODS	US	½
MEGAFOOD OPTIMUM FOODS	US	1½
MEGAFOOD WOMEN OVER 40 DAILYFOODS	US	2
MEGAFOOD WOMEN'S DAILYFOODS	US	1
MEGAFOOD WOMEN'S ONE DAILY DAILYFOODS	US	0
MELALEUCA VITALITY FOR MEN	US	1
MELALEUCA VITALITY FOR WOMEN	US	1
MELALEUCA VITALITY GOLD FOR MEN	US	2
MELALEUCA VITALITY GOLD FOR WOMEN	US	2
MELALEUCA VITALITY PACK FOR MEN	US	1
MELALEUCA VITALITY PACK FOR WOMEN	US	1
MEMBER'S MARK COMPLETE MULTI	US	0
MEMBER'S MARK MATURE MULTI	US	½
METABOLIC MAINTENANCE BASIC MAINTENANCE WITH IRON	US	1½
METABOLIC MAINTENANCE BASIC MAINTENANCE WITHOUT IRON	US	2
METABOLIC MAINTENANCE MEN'S MAINTENANCE	US	2½
METABOLIC MAINTENANCE MULTI-VITAMIN POWDER	US	1½
METABOLIC MAINTENANCE THE BIG ONE WITH IRON	US	1½
METABOLIC MAINTENANCE THE BIG ONE WITHOUT IRON	US	2
METABOLIC MAINTENANCE WOMEN'S MAINTENANCE WITH IRON	US	2
METABOLIC MAINTENANCE WOMEN'S MAINTENANCE WITHOUT IRON	US	2½
METAGENICS MULTIGENICS	US	3
METAGENICS MULTIGENICS INTENSIVE CARE	US	3½
METAGENICS MULTIGENICS INTENSIVE CARE (WITHOUT IRON)	US	3½
METAGENICS MULTIGENICS WITHOUT IRON	US	3½
MHP ACTIVITE SPORT	US	2½
MICHAEL'S ACTIVE SENIOR TABS	US	2½
MICHAEL'S FOR MEN	US	2½
MICHAEL'S FOR WOMEN	US	2½
MICHAEL'S JUST ONE	US	2
MIRACLE 2000 TOTAL BODY NUTRITION	US	2
MMS PRO PREVENTAMINS IRON FREE	US	3½
MODUCARE MULTI-MUNE	US	1
MOLECULAR BIOLOGICS ALLERVIMIN	US	1½
MOLECULAR BIOLOGICS BIO-NATURALVITE	US	1
MOLECULAR BIOLOGICS DERMA-VITES	US	1½
MOLECULAR BIOLOGICS FRUIT COLLOIDAL MINERAL & VITAMIN ELIXIR	US	1

SINGLE Product Name	Country	# of Stars
MOLECULAR BIOLOGICS LIQUI-VIMIN	US	½
MORE THAN A MULTIPLE	US	2½
MORE THAN A MULTIPLE FOR MEN	US	3
MORE THAN A MULTIPLE FOR WOMEN	US	2½
MORE THAN A MULTIPLE IRON FREE/VEGETARIAN	US	3
MOUNTAIN NATURALS OF VERMONT MEN'S SUPERIOR	US	3½
MOUNTAIN NATURALS OF VERMONT SENIOR SUPERIOR	US	3½
MOUNTAIN NATURALS OF VERMONT SUPERIOR MULTI AGE POWDER	US	4
MOUNTAIN NATURALS OF VERMONT WOMEN'S SUPERIOR	US	3½
MOUNTAIN PEAK NUTRITIONALS ENERGY FORMULA	US	2½
MOUNTAIN PEAK NUTRITIONALS ULTRA HIGH	US	3
MULTISURE FOR MEN	CA	2
MULTISURE FOR MEN 50+	CA	2
MULTISURE FOR WOMEN	CA	2
MULTISURE FOR WOMEN 50+	CA	2½
MYADEC PROFESSIONAL FORMULA	US	0
N.V. PERRICONE, M.D. PHYSICIAN'S SUPER ANTIOXIDANT	US	1½
NATROL MY FAVORITE MULTIPLE (ORIGINAL)	US	2½
NATROL MY FAVORITE MULTIPLE ENERGIZER	US	1
NATURA SELECT ADULT FOOD-BASED MULTIVITAMIN	CA/US	1
NATURA SELECT BASIC ADULT MULTI	CA/US	½
NATURA SELECT FOOD BASED MEN'S MULTI	CA/US	1½
NATURA SELECT FOOD BASED WOMEN'S MULTI	CA/US	1½
NATURAL FACTORS HI POTENCY MULTI	CA	2
NATURAL FACTORS MEN'S MULTISTART	US	3
NATURAL FACTORS MULTI FLOW ORAL CHELATION FORMULA	CA	3½
NATURAL FACTORS MULTISTART	CA	1½
NATURAL FACTORS MULTISTART MEN'S 50+	CA	3
NATURAL FACTORS MULTISTART WOMEN'S	CA	3½
NATURAL FACTORS MULTISTART WOMEN'S 45+	CA	3½
NATURAL FACTORS SUPER MULTI IRON FREE	CA	1½
NATURAL FACTORS SUPER MULTI PLUS IRON	CA	1½
NATURAL FACTORS ULTRA MULTI PLUS	CA	2
NATURAL FACTORS WELLBETX	CA	3
NATURAL FACTORS WOMEN'S MULTISTART	US	3½
NATURAL FACTORS WOMEN'S PLUS MULTISTART	US	3
NATURAL NUTRITION ACTIVE MEN'S	US	2½
NATURAL NUTRITION ACTIVE WOMAN'S	US	2½
NATURAL NUTRITION LIFE ESSENTIALS	US	2½
NATURAL NUTRITION ULTRA VMT	US	2½
NATURAL NUTRITION VI-MIN	US	2½
NATURAL NUTRITION VITA SUPER	US	1½
NATURAL NUTRITION VITA-MIN 75	US	2½
NATURAL NUTRITION VITA-MIN 75 NO IRON	US	2½
NATURALLY PREFERRED 75 COMPLETE	US	2
NATURALLY PREFERRED LIFE MULTI COMPLETE	US	2
NATURALLY PREFERRED MEN'S MULTI	US	2½
NATURALLY PREFERRED NUTRI-MAX	US	2
NATURALLY PREFERRED ONE DAILY MULTI	US	½
NATURALLY PREFERRED VITA MAX	US	2

SINGLE Product Name	Country	# of Stars
Naturally Preferred Women's Multi	US	2
Nature Made Adult Multivitamin Chewable	US	½
Nature Made Essential 50+	US	½
Nature Made Essential Balance	US	0
Nature Made Essential Daily	US	0
Nature Made Essential Man	US	½
Nature Made Essential Mega	US	1
Nature Made Essential Woman	US	½
Nature Made Multi 50+	US	½
Nature Made Multi Complete	US	0
Nature Made Multi Daily	US	0
Nature Made Multi For Her	US	0
Nature Made Multi For Her 50+	US	½
Nature Made Multi For Him	US	½
Nature Made Multi For Him 50+	US	½
Nature Made Multi Max	US	1
Nature's Answer Liquid Multiple Vitamins & Liquid Multiple Minerals	US	2
Nature's Best Tr Mega 100	US	2
Nature's Best Tr Mega 50	US	1½
Nature's Blend Mega Multivitamin With Minerals	US	1
Nature's Blend Multi-vitamin With Minerals	US	0
Nature's Blend Theratrum Complete	US	0
Nature's Bounty Multi-day Womens	US	0
Nature's Bounty Ultra Man	US	2
Nature's Bounty Ultra Woman	US	2
Nature's Bounty Weight Trim	US	½
Nature's Harmony Adult Chewable	CA	1
Nature's Harmony High Potency One Per Day	CA	?
Nature's Harmony Superior One Per Day Iron Free	CA	1
Nature's Life E-z Vite Multiple	US	1
Nature's Life Full Spectrum Antioxidant Soft Multi	US	3
Nature's Life Green Multi	US	2
Nature's Life One Daily Multiple	US	1½
Nature's Life Soft Gelatin Multiple	US	2
Nature's Life Ultra Mega Vite	US	2
Nature's Life Vegetarian Green Multi	US	2
Nature's Life Vegetarian Mega-vita-min	US	1½
Nature's Life Vegetarian Super Mega Vite	US	1½
Nature's Plus Adult's Chewable	US	1
Nature's Plus Nutri-genic	US	2
Nature's Plus Regeneration Liquid Sunshine	US	2
Nature's Plus Regeneration Soft Gels	US	3
Nature's Plus Source Of Life Adult's Chewable Wafers	US	1½
Nature's Plus Source Of Life Liquid	US	2
Nature's Plus Source Of Life Men Liquid	US	2½
Nature's Plus Source Of Life Tablets/capsules	US	2
Nature's Plus Source Of Life Women	US	2½
Nature's Plus Source Of Life Women Liquid	US	2½
Nature's Plus Ultra I	US	2
Nature's Plus Ultra II	US	2

SINGLE Product Name	Country	# of Stars
Nature's Plus Ultra Juice	US	1
Nature's Plus Ultra Source Of Life	US	2½
Nature's Plus Ultra Source Of Life No Iron	US	2½
Nature's Sunshine Super Supplemental Without Iron	US	2
Nature's Sunshine Vitawave	US	2
Nature's Valley Women's Formula	US	2
Nature's Way Alive! Drink Mix Powder	US	3
Nature's Way Alive! Tablets With Iron	US	2½
Nature's Way Alive! Vcaps/tablets, No Iron Added	US	3
Nature's Way Completia Energy	CA	1½
Nature's Way Completia Energy Plus Iron	CA	1
Nature's Way Completia Ultra Energy (Iron-free)	US	2
Nature's Way Completia Ultra Energy Multivitamin	US	2
Nature's Way Daily Two Multi Iron Free	US	3
Nature's Way Multi Vitamin Iron-free	US	3½
Nature's Way Multi Vitamin With Iron	US	3
Nature's Way Once Daily Multi	US	2
New Roots Herbal Multi-max	CA	3
New Roots Herbal Multi-max Immune	CA	4½
New Roots Herbal Phytomax	CA	1½
New Vision Juicepower Fruit/vegetable Caps	US	1
Neways Maximol Solutions	US	0
Neways Prozinger	US	1½
Newchapter Every Man	CA	1½
Newchapter Everyone's Multiple	CA	1
Newchapter Only One	CA	1
Newchapter Organics Every Man	US	1½
Newchapter Organics Every Man II	US	1½
Newchapter Organics Every Man II	CA	1½
Newchapter Organics Every Man's One Daily	CA	1
Newchapter Organics Every Woman	US	1
Newchapter Organics Every Woman II	US	1
Newchapter Organics Every Woman's One Daily	CA	1
Newchapter Organics Every Woman's One Daily	US	1
Newchapter Organics Only One	US	1
Newchapter Organics Tiny Tabs Multi	US	½
Newchapter Tiny Tabs Multiple	CA	½
Nf Formulas, Inc. Women's Formula	US	2½
Nf Formulas, Inc. Women's Formula Without Iron	US	2½
Nhk Laboratories Multi-vitamin And Mineral	US	½
Nhk Laboratories Multi-vitamin And Mineral With Lutein	US	½
Nhk Laboratories Senior Multi-vitamin And Mineral	US	½
Nikken Kenzen	US	2
North American Pharmacal Polyvite A & Phytocal A	US	2
North American Pharmacal Polyvite AB & Phytocal AB	US	2
North American Pharmacal Polyvite B & Phytocal B	US	1½
North American Pharmacal Polyvite O & Phytocal O	US	1½
Now Adam	US	2½
Now Daily Vits	US	1
Now Eco-green Multi	US	3

SINGLE Product Name	Country	# of Stars
Now Eve	US	2½
Now Special One	US	1½
Now Special Two	CA/US	2
Now Vit-min 100	US	2½
Now Vit-min 75+ Iron Free	US	2
Now Vit-min Caps	US	2½
Nsi (Neutraceutical Sciences Institute) Synergy Basic Version 2	US	3
Nsi (Neutraceutical Sciences Institute) Synergy Men's Version 2	US	5
Nsi (Neutraceutical Sciences Institute) Synergy Version 9	US	4½
Nsi (Neutraceutical Sciences Institute) Synergy Women's Version 4	US	4½
Nu-life Gourmet Chewables Multiple	CA	1½
Nu-life The Legend	CA	2½
Nu-life The Legend High Stress/activity For Men	CA	2½
Nu-life The Legend High Stress/activity For Women	CA	2
Nu-life The Legend Max Stress/activity For Men	CA	2½
Nu-life The Legend Max Stress/activity For Women	CA	2½
Nu-life Ultimate One For Men 50 Plus	CA	2
Nu-life Ultimate One For Men Active	CA	2½
Nu-life Ultimate One For Men Adult	CA	2
Nu-life Ultimate One For Women 50 Plus	CA	2
Nu-life Ultimate One For Women Active	CA	2
Nu-life Ultimate One Right Weight	CA	2½
Nu-life Ultimate One Women Adult	CA	2
Nutra Perfect Vitaperfect	US	1½
Nutra Therapeutics All-in-one	CA/US	2
Nutrametrix Multivitamins & Multiminerals With Iron	US	1
Nutrametrix Multivitamins & Multiminerals Without Iron	US	1
Nutri-betics Nutra Balance For Men	CA	2½
Nutricare Nutridaily	US	3
Nutricare Prime Greens	US	½
Nutricare Prime Greens Capsules	US	½
Nutricology Multi-vi-min	US	1½
Nutricology Multi-vi-min Without Copper & Iron	US	2
Nutriex Health	US	3½
Nutriex Sport	US	4
Nutrilite Daily	US	½
Nutrina Athlete Formula	US	2
Nutrina Champion Formula	US	2½
Nutrina Marathon Formula	US	2½
Nutrina Mega Greens	US	2
Nutrina Vitamax Powder	US	2
Nutrina Vitamax Tablets	US	1½
Nutrition Dynamics Balanced Vita-plus-min	US	3
Nutrition Dynamics Day Start & Day End Essentials	US	3½
Nutrition Dynamics Iodine Free "Vegi" Formula	US	2½
Nutrition Dynamics Multi-vitasorb	US	0
Nutrition Dynamics Ultra Fem	US	3
Nutrition Dynamics Ultra Vitaplex	US	1½
Nutrition House Men's Multi Extra	CA	2½
Nutrition House Multi-vitamin Extra	CA	1½

SINGLE Product Name	Country	# of Stars
Nutrition House Multi-vitamin Extra Iron Free	CA	2
Nutrition House Women's Multi Extra	CA	2½
Nutrition Now Adult Formula	US	0
Nutrition Now Multi Earth Force	US	2½
Nutrivene-d Advanced Formula Daily Supplement	US	2½
Nutrivene-d Full Spectrum Formula	US	3
Nutri-west Core Level Health Reserve	US	2½
Nutri-west Multi Complex	US	1
Nutri-west Multibalance For Men	US	1½
Nutri-west Multibalance For Women	US	1½
Nutri-west Total Female	US	0
Nutri-west Total Male	US	½
Ola Loa Super Multi (Tropical)	US	3
Ola Loa Super Multi (Orange)	US	3
Olay Complete 50+ Multivitamin	US	½
Olay Complete Multivitamin	US	½
Olay Complete Woman's Multivitamin	US	½
Olay Complete Woman's Multivitamin 50+	US	½
Olympian Labs Vita Vitamin	US	2½
Olympian Labs Vita-one	US	2½
Omnilife Magnus	US	½
Omnitrition Omni IV	US	½
Omnitrition Shield Antioxidant	US	1½
One A Day 50 Plus	US	½
One A Day Active	US	½
One A Day Adults	CA	0
One A Day Adults 50+	CA	½
One A Day Carbsmart	US	½
One A Day Cholesterol Plus	US	½
One A Day Maximum	US	0
One A Day Men's	CA	½
One A Day Men's Health Formula	US	½
One A Day Weight Smart	CA	1
One A Day Weight Smart	US	1
One A Day Women's	CA	0
One A Day Women's	US	0
Onesource 50 Plus	US	½
Onesource Advanced Formula	US	½
Onesource Men's	US	2
Onesource Micro	US	½
Onesource Pure Performance	US	½
Onesource Women's	US	2
Optimox Androvite For Men	US	3
Optimox Gynovite Plus	US	2
Optimox Optivite Pmt For Women	US	2½
Oregon Health Multi-guard With CoQ$_{10}$	US	3½
Oregon Health Women's Multiple	US	3
Organika One Daily	CA	1½
Origin Complete Multi-vitamin & Mineral	US	0
Original Medicine Nutrasyn	US	2

SINGLE Product Name	Country	# of Stars
Ortho Molecular Products Alpha Base Capsules	US	4
Ortho Molecular Products Alpha Base Capsules Without Iron	US	4½
Ortho Molecular Products Alpha Base Capsules Without Iron Or Copper	US	4½
Ortho Molecular Products Alpha Base Tablets	US	4½
Pataki Usa 2001 Formula	US	1½
Pataki Usa 2101 Formula	US	1
Performance Labs Vitalert	US	½
Personnelle Complete	CA	0
Personnelle Forte	CA	0
Personnelle Natura Senior	CA	½
Personnelle Senior	CA	½
Personnelle Superia	CA	½
Peter Gillham's Natural Vitality Liquid Organic Life Vitamins	US	2
Pharmacist's Ultimate Health Man's Ultimate Formula	US	3
Pharmacist's Ultimate Health Woman's Ultimate Formula	US	3
Pharmanex Life Essentials	CA	1
Pharmanex Life Essentials	US	1
Pharmassure Men's Biomultiple	US	1½
Pharmassure Women's Biomultiple	US	1½
Pharmaton Ginsana Gold Formula	US	½
Physician Formulas Multivit-Rx	US	2
Phytobec	CA	½
Phytopharmica Clinical Nutrients For 45-plus Women	US	4
Phytopharmica Clinical Nutrients For 50-plus Men	US	4
Phytopharmica Clinical Nutrients For Men	US	3½
Phytopharmica Clinical Nutrients For Women	US	3½
Pioneer Chewable	US	2½
Pioneer Vegetarian 1+ Vitamin Mineral	US	3
Plante Gummi 50+	CA/US	½
Platinum Active Easymulti Plus For Men	CA	3
Platinum Active Easymulti Plus For Women	CA	3
Platinum Easymulti	CA	1
Platinum Megavita Minerals With Hempseed Oil	CA	½
Platinum Super Easymulti Plus For Men 45+	CA	3
Platinum Super Easymulti Plus For Women 45+	CA	3
Prairie Naturals Multi-force Powder	CA	2
Prairie Naturals Multi-force	CA	3
Prevention Diabetic Support	US	2
Prevention Dieter's Complete	CA	2½
Prevention Dieter's Complete	US	2
Prevention For Men	CA/US	2½
Prevention For Men 50 Plus	CA	2½
Prevention For Men 50 Plus	US	2½
Prevention For Women	CA	2½
Prevention For Women	US	2½
Prevention For Women 50 Plus	CA	2½
Prevention For Women 50 Plus	US	2½
Pro Health Multiple One	US	2½
Pro Health Super Multiple II	US	2

SINGLE Product Name	Country	# of Stars
Pro Health Super Multiple Without Iron	US	3
Pro Image Pro Vitamin Complete	US	0
Pro-caps Laboratories Cholox	US	3
Professional Health Products Multidyn	CA	1½
Professional Health Products Multi-pro	CA	2½
Progressive For Active Men	CA	3
Progressive For Active Women	CA	3
Progressive For Adult Men	CA	2½
Progressive For Adult Women	CA	2½
Progressive For Men Over 50	CA	3
Progressive For Women Over 50	CA	3
Prothera Lda Multi-vitamin & Lda Trace Mineral Complex	US	2½
Prothera Multithera 1	US	4
Prothera Multithera 2	US	3½
Prothera Vitaprime	US	2½
Pure Advantage Womens Multiple	US	2
Pure Encapsulations Nutrient 280	US	1½
Pure Encapsulations Nutrient 950	US	3
Pure Encapsulations Nutrient 950 With Nac	US	3
Pure Encapsulations Nutrient 950 Without Copper & Iron	US	3
Pure Encapsulations Nutrient 950 Without Copper, Iron & Iodine	US	3½
Pure Encapsulations Nutrient 950 Without Iron	US	3½
Pure Encapsulations Ultranutrient	US	4
Pure Essence Labs Life Essence Powder	US	4
Pure Essence Labs Life Essence Tablets	US	4
Pure Essence Labs One'n'only	US	2
Puritan's Pride Daily 3 Caps	US	2½
Puritan's Pride Formula 100	US	2
Puritan's Pride Green Source	US	2
Puritan's Pride Green Source Iron Free	US	2½
Puritan's Pride Mega Vita Gel	US	2
Puritan's Pride Mega Vita Min	US	2
Puritan's Pride Mega Vita Min For Seniors	US	2
Puritan's Pride Mega Vita Min For Women	US	2
Puritan's Pride Mega Vita Min For Women Iron Free	US	2
Puritan's Pride Mega Vita Min Iron Free	US	2
Puritan's Pride Multi-day Plus Minerals	US	0
Puritan's Pride Potent 75 Super Vm	US	1½
Puritan's Pride Puritron	US	1
Puritan's Pride Theravim-m	US	0
Puritan's Pride Ultra Man 75	US	3
Puritan's Pride Ultra Vita Man	US	2
Puritan's Pride Ultra Vita-min	US	1
Puritan's Pride Ultra Vita-min Iron Free	US	1
Puritan's Pride Women's Exclusive Formula	US	1½
Purity Products Fizz-5 Formula	US	1
Purity Products The Perfect Multi	US	3½
Purity Products The Perfect Multi Super Greens	US	3½
Qci Nutritionals Daily Preventive #1	US	3½
Qci Nutritionals Ultra Vitality #2	US	3

SINGLE Product Name	Country	# of Stars
Qci Nutritionals Ultra Vitality #3	US	3½
Qci Nutritionals Ultra Vitality Elite	US	3½
Quest Adults	CA	1
Quest Extra Once A Day	CA	1
Quest Maximum Once A Day	CA	2½
Quest Premium Multi-cap	CA	1
Quest Premium Multi-one	CA	1½
Quest Super Once A Day	CA	1½
Radiance Green Source Iron Free	US	2½
Radiance Mega Vita Gel	US	2
Radiance Mega Vita-min Iron Free	US	2
Rainbow Light Advanced Nutritional System	US	3
Rainbow Light Advanced Nutritional System Iron-free	US	3½
Rainbow Light Complete Nutritional System	US	2½
Rainbow Light Just Once	US	1
Rainbow Light Just Once Active Senior	US	2
Rainbow Light Just Once Iron-frff	US	1
Rainbow Light Just Once Men's Energy	US	1½
Rainbow Light Just Once Men's One	US	1½
Rainbow Light Just Once Women's One	US	1½
Rainbow Light Master Nutrient System Plus	US	1½
Rainbow Light Rejuvenage 40+	US	4
Rainbow Light Women's Nutritional System	US	2½
Rbc Life Sciences 24seven Life Essentials	CA/US	1½
Rejuvenation Science Maximum Vitality	US	5
Relìv Classic	CA	1
Relìv Classic	US	1
Relìv Now	CA	1
Relìv Now	US	1
Resource Optisource	US	1½
Resurgex	US	1½
Resurgex Plus	US	1½
Resurgex Select	US	1
Revival Firm Foundation	US	1
Rexall Complete	CA	0
Rexall Complete For Adults 50+	CA	½
Rexall Complete Forte	CA	0
Rexall Multiple Vitamins & Minerals	CA	0
Rexall Multivitamin + Multimineral Forte	CA	0
Rexall One Tablet Daily Adult	CA	0
Rexall One Tablet Daily Adults 50+	CA	½
Rexall One Tablet Daily Women's	CA	0
Rexall One Weigh	CA	1
R-garden Vitamin Mineral Formula	US	1½
Ripple Creek Mega-100	US	2½
Ripple Creek Mega-caps 2	US	2
Ripple Creek Mega-one 75	US	1½
Rite Aid Central-vite	US	0
Rite Aid Central-vite Select	US	½
Rite Aid High Potency Multi	US	0

SINGLE Product Name	Country	# of Stars
RITE AID ONE DAILY	US	0
RITE AID ONE DAILY LOW CARB SUPPORT	US	½
RITE AID ONE DAILY MEN'S MULTI	US	½
RITE AID ONE DAILY WOMEN'S	US	0
RITE AID THERAPEUTIC M	US	0
RITE AID TRIM SUPPORT	US	½
RITE AID WHOLE SOURCE	US	½
RITE AID WHOLE SOURCE COMPLETE FORMULA FOR WOMEN	US	1½
RITE AID WHOLE SOURCE MATURE ADULT	US	1
RITE AID WHOLE SOURCE MEN	US	1
RITE AID WHOLE SOURCE WOMEN	US	1
RX VITAMINS REVITALIZE	US	3
RX VITAMINS REVITALIZE WITHOUT IRON	US	3
SAFEWAY SELECT CENTRAL-VITE	US	0
SAFEWAY SELECT CENTRAL-VITE PERFORMANCE	US	½
SAFEWAY SELECT CENTRAL-VITE SENIOR FORMULA	US	½
SAFEWAY SELECT FORMULA FORTE	CA	0
SAFEWAY SELECT FORMULA FORTE SENIOR	CA	½
SAFEWAY SELECT FORMULE POUR 50+	CA	½
SAFEWAY SELECT FORMULE POUR HOMMES	CA	½
SAFEWAY SELECT FORMULE RÉGULIÈRE	CA	0
SAFEWAY SELECT MAXIMUM ONE TABLET DAILY	US	0
SAFEWAY SELECT MULTIVITAMIN & MINERAL	US	0
SAFEWAY SELECT ONE TABLET DAILY DIETER'S SUPPORT FORMULA	US	1
SAFEWAY SELECT ONE TABLET DAILY MEN'S HEALTH	US	½
SAFEWAY SELECT ONE TABLET DAILY WOMEN'S	US	0
SAFEWAY SELECT SUPER MEN'S MULTIVITAMIN	US	1½
SAFEWAY SELECT SUPER WOMEN'S MULTIVITAMIN	US	2
SAFEWAY SELECT WEIGHT-CONSCIOUS	CA	1
SAFEWAY SELECT WOMEN'S FORMULA	CA	0
SANGSTER'S CHOICE APEX	CA	½
SANGSTER'S CHOICE APEX	US	½
SANGSTER'S DAILY CHOICE	CA/US	1
SANGSTER'S MEN'S CHOICE	US	2½
SANGSTER'S MULTI VITAMIN	CA	1½
SANGSTER'S MULTI VITAMIN	US	1½
SANGSTER'S SENIOR'S CHOICE	US	2
SANGSTER'S VEGE CHOICE	US	2
SANGSTER'S WOMEN'S CHOICE	US	2
SAV-ON OSCO ONE DAILY MAXIMUM	US	0
SCHIFF PRIME YEARS	US	1
SCHIFF SINGLE DAY	US	2
SCHIFF VEGETARIAN MULTIPLE	US	½
SCHWARZBEIN INSTITUTE ULTRA PREVENTIVE III (CAPSULES)	US	3
SCHWARZBEIN INSTITUTE ULTRA PREVENTIVE III (TABLETS)	US	4
SELEKTA MULTI II'S WITH COPPER & IRON	CA	2
SELEKTA MULTI'S WITHOUT COPPER & IRON	CA	2
SELEKTA SELEKTA-CLEAR	CA	4½
SEROYAL SUPER ORTI VITE	CA	2½
SHAKLEE ADVANCED FORMULA VITA-LEA	CA	1

SINGLE PRODUCT NAME	COUNTRY	# OF STARS
SHAKLEE VITA-LEA GOLD WITH VITAMIN K	US	1½
SHAKLEE VITA-LEA GOLD WITHOUT VITAMIN K	US	1½
SHAKLEE VITA-LEA WITH IRON	US	1
SHAKLEE VITA-LEA WITHOUT IRON	US	1
SISU MINI VITS	CA	1½
SISU MULTI ACTIVE	CA	2
SISU MULTI ACTIVE WOMAN	CA	2
SISU MULTI-VI-MIN	CA	1
SISU ONLY ONE	CA	1½
SISU ONLY ONE IRON FREE	CA	1½
SISU VEGI MINS	CA	2½
SOLARAY MEN'S GOLDEN MULTI-VITA-MIN	US	2
SOLARAY MULTI-VITA MEGA MINERAL MULTI-VITA-MIN	US	2½
SOLARAY ONCE DAILY HIGH ENERGY	US	1½
SOLARAY ONCE DAILY HIGH ENERGY IRON FREE	US	1½
SOLARAY ONCE DAILY HIGH ENERGY SOFTGEL	CA	1½
SOLARAY ONCE DAILY IRON FREE	US	1
SOLARAY PROVIDE	US	2
SOLARAY PROVIDE IRON FREE	US	2½
SOLARAY SPECTRO 3	US	3
SOLARAY SPECTRO 3 IRON FREE	US	3
SOLARAY SPECTRO MULTI-VITA-MIN	US	3
SOLARAY SPECTRO MULTI-VITA-MIN	CA	2
SOLARAY SPECTRO MULTI-VITA-MIN IRON FREE	US	2½
SOLARAY SPECTRO MULTI-VITA-MIN IRON FREE	CA	2½
SOLARAY SPECTRO SMOOTHIE ONCE DAILY	US	3
SOLARAY THREE DAILY SUPER ENERGY	US	2½
SOLARAY THREE DAILY SUPER ENERGY IRON FREE	US	3
SOLARAY TWICE DAILY IRON FREE	US	2½
SOLARAY TWICE DAILY MULTI ENERGY	US	2
SOLARAY TWICE DAILY MULTI ENERGY IRON FREE	US	2½
SOLARAY VEGETARIAN SPECTRO MULTI-VITA-MIN	US	3
SOLARAY VITAPRIME FOR MEN	US	2½
SOLARAY VITAPRIME FOR WOMEN	US	2½
SOLARAY WOMEN'S GOLDEN MULTI-VITA-MIN	US	2½
SOLGAR EARTH SOURCE MULTI-NUTRIENT	US	2
SOLGAR FEMALE MULTIPLE	US	3
SOLGAR FORMULA VM-2000	US	2
SOLGAR FORMULA VM-75	US	2
SOLGAR FORMULA VM-75 IRON-FREE	US	2
SOLGAR FORMULA VM-PRIME	US	2
SOLGAR MALE MULTIPLE	US	3½
SOLGAR NATURVITE	US	1½
SOLGAR OMNIUM	US	3
SOLGAR OMNIUM IRON-FREE	US	3½
SOLGAR SOLOVITE IRON FREE	US	1
SOLGAR VEGETARIAN MULTIPLE	US	1½
SOMALIFE SOMAVIT PLUS	CA/US	2½
SONERGY MEGA PLAN	US	1½
SONERGY ONE DAILY MULTIPLE WITH IRON	US	0

SINGLE Product Name	Country	# of Stars
Source Naturals Élan Vitàl Multiple	US	5
Source Naturals Life Defense	US	3
Source Naturals Life Force Multiple	US	5
Source Naturals Ultra Multiple	US	2
Source Naturals Wellness Multiple	US	4
Spring Valley Naturally Complete Multivitamin	US	½
Spring Valley Sentury-vite	US	½
Standard Process Catalyn	US	0
Standard Process Immunoplex	US	½
Sundown Complete 50+	US	½
Sundown Complete Daily	US	½
Sundown Complete Multi 50+	US	½
Sundown Complete Ultra	US	1
Sundown Complete Women's	US	½
Sundown Sunvite	US	0
Sunmark Complete Advanced	US	0
Sunmark Complete Senior	US	½
Sunmark Multiple Vitamins Women's	US	0
Sunmark Therapeutic-m	US	½
Supernutrition Longevity	US	2
Supernutrition Men's Blend	US	4
Supernutrition Multi Vitamin & Mineral	CA	2
Supernutrition Perfect Blend	US	3½
Supernutrition Simply One	US	2
Supernutrition Simply One Men	US	2
Supernutrition Simply One Women	US	2
Supralife Formula Plus	US	2½
Supralife Maxum Essentials	US	2½
Supralife Total Toddy	US	2
Supralife Ultra Body Toddy With Cell Shield	US	3
Swanson Active One	US	1½
Swanson Active One Without Iron	US	2
Swanson All-day Complete	US	2½
Swanson All-day Complete For Seniors Without Iron	US	3
Swanson Century Formula Without Iron	US	1
Swanson High Potency Soft Multiple	US	2
Swanson High Potency Soft Multiple Iron Free	US	2½
Swanson Lee Swanson Signature Line Longevital	US	5
Swanson Ultra Whole Food	US	2½
Swiss Adult Multi One Formula	CA	2
Swiss Hi Potency Swiss One "80"	CA	2
Swiss Mega Swiss One "25"	CA	1
Swiss Slim Essentials	CA	2
Swiss Super Adult	CA	1½
Swiss Super Swiss One "50"	CA	1½
Swiss Swiss One	CA	½
Swiss Swiss Total One Men	CA	3
Swiss Swiss Total One Women	CA	2½
Swiss Total One	CA	3
Swiss Vege Multivitamin And Mineral	CA	2

SINGLE Product Name	Country	# of Stars
Symmetry Ultra Vitality	US	1
Synergy Multiple Vitamin/mineral	US	½
Target Adult Multivitamin/multimineral	US	0
Target Men's Daily Multivitamin	US	½
Target Multivitamin/multimineral	US	0
Target Multivitamin/multimineral For Adults 50+	US	½
Target Weight Sense	US	1
Target Women's Daily Multivitamin	US	0
The Greatest Vitamin In The World	US	2
The Green Turtle Bay Co. Powervites	US	1½
The Green Turtle Bay Vitamin Co. Diabetiks & Powervites	US	3
The Green Turtle Bay Vitamin Co. Maple Melts	US	1
The Synergy Company Vita Synergy For Men	US	2½
The Synergy Company Vita Synergy For Women	US	2½
Theragran-m Advanced Formula	US	½
Theragran-m Premier	US	½
Theragran-m Premier 50 Plus	US	½
Thompson Adult-plex	US	2
Thompson Coach's Formula	US	2
Thompson Mega 80	US	2
Thompson Multi Formula For Women	US	½
Thompson Multi-vitamins	US	½
Thompson Nuplex	US	½
Thompson Super Maxicaps	US	1½
Thorne Research Al's Formula	US	3½
Thorne Research Basic Nutrients I	US	3
Thorne Research Basic Nutrients II	US	3
Thorne Research Basic Nutrients III	US	3
Thorne Research Basic Nutrients III Without Copper & Iron	US	3
Thorne Research Basic Nutrients IV	US	3
Thorne Research Basic Nutrients V	US	3
Thorne Research Extra Nutrients	US	3½
Thorne Research Meta-fem	US	3½
Thorne Research Nutri-fem	US	3
Top Care Complete	US	0
Top Care Complete Advantage	US	½
Top Care Complete Senior	US	½
Top Care Multi For Women	US	0
Top Care One Daily 50+	US	½
Top Care One Daily Dieter's Support Formula	US	0
Top Care One Daily Maximum	US	0
Top Care One Daily Men's	US	½
Top Care One Daily Women's	US	0
Total Multivitamin	US	½
Totalone Supermulti	US	½
Trace Minerals Complete Foods Multi	US	2½
Trace Minerals Electro-vita-min	US	1½
Trace Minerals Electro-vita-min (New & Improved)	US	1½
Trace Minerals Immunomax	US	½
Trace Minerals Liquid Multi Vita-mineral	US	2

SINGLE PRODUCT NAME		COUNTRY	# OF STARS
TRACE MINERALS MAXI MULTI		US	1
TRC NUTRITIONAL LABORATORIES FEMALE BASIC MULTIPLE		US	1
TRC NUTRITIONAL LABORATORIES LIQUID LIFE		US	2½
TRC NUTRITIONAL LABORATORIES MALE BASIC MULTIPLE		US	1½
TRC NUTRITIONAL LABORATORIES VAST VITALITY		US	1½
TRIVITA DAILY MEN		US	1½
TRIVITA DAILY WOMEN		US	1½
TRIVITA VITADAILY AM/PM		US	2
TROPHIC COMPLETE		CA	3
TROPHIC MULTIPLE VITAMINS & MINERALS		CA	1
TROPHIC SELECT		CA	2
TROPICAL OASIS MULTIPLE VITAMIN/MINERAL		US	½
TROPICAL OASIS TROPICAL PLUS		US	1½
TRUESTAR HEALTH TRUEBASIC		CA	5 GOLD
TRULY CENTURY PLUS		CA	0
TRULY CENTURY PREMIUM		CA	½
TRULY CENTURY SILVER		CA	½
TRULY WEIGHT ONE		CA	1
TWINLAB DAILY ONE CAPS WITH IRON		US	1½
TWINLAB DAILY ONE CAPS WITHOUT IRON		US	1½
TWINLAB DUALTABS		US	2
TWINLAB FOOD-BASED ULTRA DAILY		US	1
TWINLAB MEN'S ULTRA DAILY		US	2½
TWINLAB WOMEN'S ULTRA DAILY		US	2½
ULTIMA FOR MEN		US	1
ULTIMA FOR WOMEN		US	½
ULTIMATE NUTRITION SUPER COMPLETE		US	3½
UNICAP M DIETARY SUPPLEMENT		US	0
UNICAP SR. DIETARY SUPPLEMENT		US	0
UNICITY BIOS LIFE 2 ORIGINAL		US	0
UNICITY COREHEALTH FOR MEN		US	2
UNICITY COREHEALTH FOR WOMEN		US	2
UNICITY LIFEHEALTH ON THE GO		US	1
UNIVERSAL NUTRITION GENESIS		CA	2
UNIVERSAL NUTRITION MEGA EDGE		CA	2
USANA HEALTH SCIENCES ESSENTIALS	*EDITOR'S CHOICE*	CA	5 GOLD
USANA HEALTH SCIENCES ESSENTIALS	*AWARD WINNERS*	US	5 GOLD
VÄXA DAILY ESSENTIALS		US	2
VEGLIFE IRON FREE MULTIVEG ENERGY		US	3
VEGLIFE SPECTRO VEG HIGH ENERGY		US	2½
VEGLIFE VEGAN ONE MULTIPLE		CA/US	2
VIACTIV MULTI-VITAMIN		US	0
VICON-C HIGH POTENCY MULTIVITAMIN/MINERAL		US	0
VIRTUVITES IRON-FREE VITA-MIN 75		US	2½
VISALUS NUTRI-ONE		US	1½
VISION FOR LIFE BODY FORCE		US	2
VITA-COMPLETE AA (ANTI-AGING)		CA/US	½
VITA-COMPLETE VITA-COMPLETE 29		CA/US	0
VITAL NUTRIENTS MINIMAL AND ESSENTIAL		US	2
VITAL NUTRIENTS MULTI NUTRIENTS V		US	2½

SINGLE Product Name	Country	# of Stars
Vital Nutrients Multi-nutrients II	US	3
Vital Nutrients Multi-nutrients III	US	3
Vital Nutrients Multi-nutrients IV	US	2½
Vital Nutrients Multi-nutrients No Iron Or Iodine	US	3½
Vital Nutrients Multi-nutrients Veg Caps No Iron Or Iodine	US	3
Vital Nutrients Multi-nutrients With Iron And Iodine	US	3
Vitalert	US	½
Vitality New Generation	US	2
Vitality Products Multi-vitamins And Minerals	US	2
Vitality Products Two-a-day	US	1½
Vitamin Power Mega Multiple 85	US	1
Vitamin Power Power Source 100	US	2
Vitamin Power Superfem Multiple	US	1½
Vitamin Power Super-vite	US	1
Vitamin Power Ultra Multi 90 Plus	US	2
Vitamin Power Vita-max	US	1
Vitamin Research Products Extend Core	US	3
Vitamin Research Products Extend Liquid	US	2½
Vitamin Research Products Extend One	US	2
Vitamin Research Products Extend Plus	US	4½
Vitamin Research Products Optimum 18	US	5
Vitamin Research Products Optimum 6	US	4
Vitamin Research Products Optimum D	US	3½
Vitamin Research Products Optimum Silver	US	3
Vitamin Research Products Women's Essentials	US	3
Vitamin Shoppe Daily 3 Complete	US	3
Vitamin Shoppe From The Earth (Without Iron)	US	2½
Vitamin Shoppe Life Essentials Multi	US	4½
Vitamin Shoppe Mega-vites 75	US	2
Vitamin Shoppe One Daily	US	1½
Vitamin Shoppe Ultimate Man	US	2
Vitamin Shoppe Ultimate Woman	US	2
Vitamin Shoppe Ultimate Woman No Iron	US	2
Vitamin World Abc Plus	US	0
Vitamin World Daily 3 Caps	US	2½
Vitamin World Green Source	US	2½
Vitamin World Mega Vita Gel	US	2
Vitamin World Mega Vita Min For Seniors	US	2
Vitamin World Mega Vita Min For Women	US	2
Vitamin World Mega Vita Min For Women With Iron	US	2
Vitamin World Mega Vita-min	US	2
Vitamin World Mega Vita-min Iron Free	US	2
Vitamin World Nutri-100 Gold	US	2
Vitamin World Theravim-m	US	0
Vitamin World Ultra Vita Man	US	2
Vitamin World Ultra Vita-min	US	½
Vitamin World Ultra Vita-min Iron Free	US	1
Vitaminerals Combadult	US	1
Vitaminerals Combadult M	US	1
Vitaplen Complete	US	½

SINGLE Product Name	Country	# of Stars
Vitaplex Total One Daily	CA	2
Vitasmart Advanced Formula Complete	US	0
Vitasmart Carb-vantage	US	½
Vitasmart Century Advantage	US	½
Vitasmart Complete Senior	US	½
Vitasmart Daily Diet Support	US	1
Vitasmart Hi Potency Complete	US	0
Vitasmart Maximum	US	0
Vitasmart Men's Health Formula	US	½
Vitasmart Men's Premium Multivitamin	US	1½
Vitasmart Select Men's Multi	US	2
Vitasmart Select Super Multi 50+	US	½
Vitasmart Select Women's Multi	US	1½
Vitasmart Women's	US	0
Vitazan Multi-power	CA	3
Vitosophy	US	1
Viva Life Science Dailyguard	US	2
Viva Life Science Liquiguard	US	2½
Viva Life Science Viva For Life	US	1
Walgreens A Thru Z	US	0
Walgreens A Thru Z Advantage	US	½
Walgreens A Thru Z Select	US	½
Walgreens One Daily 50 Plus	US	½
Walgreens One Daily Men's	US	½
Walgreens One Daily Women's	US	0
Walgreens One Daily Women's 50 Plus	US	½
Walgreens Super Aytinal For Active Adults	US	0
Walgreens Super Aytinal For Adults 50 Plus	US	½
Walgreens Therapeutic M	US	½
Walgreens Ultrachoice Adult	US	½
Walgreens Ultrachoice Mature	US	1
Wampole Adult Chewable	CA	½
Wampole Hsn Formula Women's	CA	½
Watkins Super Multi	CA	1½
Watkins Superfood Multiple	US	1½
Weil Daily Multivitamin For Optimum Health	US	2
Weil Daily Multivitamin Formula	CA	2
Wellbetx Complete Diabetic	CA	3
Wellness International Network Phyto-vite	US	2½
Wellness Resources Daily Energy	US	2½
Westcoast Naturals Multi-plus	CA	½
Western Family Active Women 50+	US	½
Western Family Complete Advanced	US	0
Western Family Complete Premium	US	½
Western Family Complete Senior Formula	US	½
Western Family Daily Diet Support	US	1
Western Family Multi Vitamins With Minerals	CA	½
Western Family Multra	CA	½
Western Family Multra 50+	CA	1
Western Family Multra With Iron	CA	½

SINGLE Product Name	Country	# of Stars
WESTERN FAMILY ONE DAILY MAXIMUM	US	0
WESTERN FAMILY ONE DAILY WOMEN'S	US	0
WESTERN FAMILY THERAPEUTIC M	US	½
WHEATIES MULTIVITAMIN	US	1
WILD OATS BASIC MULTI	US	½
WILD OATS FOOD ORIGINS MEN'S PRIME PLUS MULTI-VITAMIN	US	1½
WILD OATS FOOD ORIGINS MULTI-VITAMIN ONE	US	½
WILD OATS FOOD ORIGINS WOMEN'S PRIME PLUS MULTI-VITAMIN	US	1½
WILD OATS IRON FREE MULTI CAPS	US	2
WILD OATS IRON FREE ULTIMATE ONE	US	2
WILD OATS LIFE MULTI COMPLETE	US	2
WILD OATS MULTI-VITAMIN ONE	US	0
WILD OATS ULTIMATE ONE	US	2
WILD OATS ULTIMATE TWO	US	2
WILD OATS ULTIMATE VEGETARIAN MULTI	US	2
WIN FUEL MEN'S FORMULA	US	½
WIN FUEL WOMEN'S FORMULA	US	0
WOMEN'S INTERNATIONAL PHARMACY NUTRI-WOMAN	US	2½
WOMEN'S INTERNATIONAL PHARMACY OSTEOEMPHASIS	US	2½
XTEND-LIFE TOTAL BALANCE MEN'S PLUS	NZ/US	2½
XTEND-LIFE TOTAL BALANCE UNISEX	NZ/US	2½
XTEND-LIFE TOTAL BALANCE WOMEN'S PLUS	NZ/US	3
XYMOGEN ACTIVNUTRIENTS	US	3
XYMOGEN ACTIVNUTRIENTS WOMEN (WITH IRON)	US	2
XYMOGEN ACTIVNUTRIENTS WOMEN (WITHOUT IRON)	US	2
XYMOGEN INSULEAN RICE	US	1
XYMOGEN INSULEAN SOY	US	2
YOUNG AGAIN NUTRIENTS COMPLETE ONE	US	2
YOUNG AGAIN NUTRIENTS ULTRAHIGH	US	3
YOUNG AGAIN NUTRIENTS ULTRAMAN	US	2½
YOUNG AGAIN NUTRIENTS ULTRAWOMAN	US	2
ZAND HERBAL FORMULAS ZANERGY	US	2
ZIQUIN MIND & BODY TONIC	US	1½

CHAPTER 8:

COMBINATION PRODUCT RATINGS

Sorted Alphabetically by Product Name

COMBINATION Product Name	Country	# of Stars
AMERISCIENCES MEN'S MASTER MULTI	US	2½
AMERISCIENCES WOMEN'S MASTER MULTI	US	2½
ARBONNE INTERNATIONAL DAILY POWER PACKS FOR MEN	US	2½
ARBONNE INTERNATIONAL DAILY POWER PACKS FOR WOMEN	US	2½
BIOX MULTI VITAMIN PACK	CA	4
BRONSON LABORATORIES DAILY NUTRIONAL PACKETS	US	1½
BRONSON LABORATORIES NUTRITIONAL PACKETS FOR ACTIVE MEN	US	1½
BRONSON LABORATORIES NUTRITIONAL PACKETS FOR ACTIVE WOMEN	US	1½
CLUB VITAMIN MEGA VITAMIN KIT	CA	1½
COLGAN INSTITUTE BASIC BODY ARMOR	US	2½
COLGAN INSTITUTE MEN'S ACTIVE PAK	US	4½
COLGAN INSTITUTE MEN'S FIRST DEFENSE PAK	US	3
COLGAN INSTITUTE MEN'S PAK	US	5
COLGAN INSTITUTE MEN'S+ 50 PAK	US	5
COLGAN INSTITUTE SPORTS PAK	US	5
COLGAN INSTITUTE WOMEN'S 50+ PAK	US	5
COLGAN INSTITUTE WOMEN'S ACTIVE PAK	US	5
COLGAN INSTITUTE WOMEN'S FIRST DEFENSE	US	3
COLGAN INSTITUTE WOMEN'S PAK	US	5
CVC 4 HEALTH UNIT PAC ORIGINAL	US	1½
CVC 4 HEALTH UNIT PAC ROYAL	US	2
CVC 4 HEALTH UNIT PAC SUPREME	US	2
CVC 4 HEALTH UNIT PAC ULTIMATE	US	3
DC (DEE CEE LABORATORIES) MEGA VITA-MIN	US	3
DOUGLAS LABORATORIES BASIC ANTIOX	US	4
DOUGLAS LABORATORIES DAD'S PACK	US	4½
DOUGLAS LABORATORIES DAILY CORE ESSENTIALS	CA	5 GOLD
DOUGLAS LABORATORIES ESSENTIAL-4 NUTRITION PACK	US	4
DOUGLAS LABORATORIES LONGEVITY SUPPORT PACK	US	5 GOLD
DOUGLAS LABORATORIES MET-A-SYN X-PACK	US	2½
DOUGLAS LABORATORIES NUTRI-PAK FOR MEN	US	4
DOUGLAS LABORATORIES NUTRI-PAK FOR WOMEN	US	4
DOUGLAS LABORATORIES OC PACK	US	4
DOUGLAS LABORATORIES ULTRA PREVENTIVE V PLUS CHEL-SUPPLEMENT PACK	US	3
DR. LARK DAILY ANSWER MULTINUTRIENT FOR WOMEN	US	3½
DR. LARK DAILY BALANCE WOMEN'S MULTINUTRIENT	US	3½
ENEREX OPTIMAL HEALTH PACK	CA	2
ENZYMATIC THERAPY ENERGY REVITALIZATION SYSTEM (CITRUS DELIGHT)	US	3½
EPIC4HEALTH PHYSICIAN'S RX COMPLETE FORMULA	US	3
EQUALINE DAILY VITAMIN PACKETS	US	2

COMBINATION PRODUCT NAME	COUNTRY	# OF STARS
FORMOR INTERNATIONAL CORE NUTRITION	US	3½
FREELIFE BASIC MINDELL PLUS	US	3
GLOBAL HEALTH TRAX BASIC FIVE	US	2
GNC MAXIMUM NUTRITION VITAPAK	US	2
GNC MEGA MEN PERFORMANCE AND VITALITY PROGRAM	US	2
GNC WOMEN'S ULTRA MEGA WELLNESS PROGRAM	US	2
GNLD INTERNATIONAL DAILY VITALITY PACK ACTIVE 40+	US	2½
GNLD INTERNATIONAL DAILY VITALITY PACK SPORTS 30	US	2½
GNLD INTERNATIONAL DAILY VITALITY PACK STRESS 30	US	2½
GREAT AMERICAN PRODUCTS MASTER HEALTH PACK	US	3½
GREAT EARTH NUTRITIONAL STARTER PACK (EXTRA STRENGTH)	US	3
GREAT EARTH NUTRITIONAL STARTER PACK (REGULAR STRENGTH)	US	2
GREAT EARTH NUTRITIONAL STARTER PACK (ULTRA STRENGTH)	US	3½
GUTHY-RENKER NUTRITION GRN VITAPOWER	US	1
HANNEN HEALTH DAILY ESSENTIALS	US	1½
HERBASWAY LABORATORIES DAILY MAINTENANCE GROUP	US	1½
HIGHLAND LABORATORIES MEN'S SPORTS PAK	US	3½
HIGHLAND LABORATORIES SUPER ATHLETE PACKS	US	3
HIGHLAND LABORATORIES WOMEN'S SPORTS PAK	US	3½
INVITE MULTI-VITAMIN	US	3
JARROW FORMULAS ALL CAPSULE HEALTH PAK	US	4
JARROW FORMULAS JARROW PAK PLUS	US	3½
JEAN CARPER'S STOP AGING NOW! ANTI-AGING POWER-PAK	US	4½
JULIAN WHITAKER, M.D. FORWARD PLUS DAILY REGIMEN	CA	4
JULIAN WHITAKER, M.D. FORWARD PLUS DAILY REGIMEN	US	4½
KIRKLAND DAILY MULTIVITAMIN PACK	US	1½
LIFE-LINE MEN'S LIFE-PACK	US	1½
LIFE-LINE TOTAL HEALTH FORMULA	US	3½
LIFE-LINE WOMEN'S LIFE-PACK	US	1
LORNA VANDERHAEGHE FEMMESSENTIALS	CA/US	4
MELALEUCA DAILY FOR LIFE TOTAL NUTRITION FOR MEN	US	2
MELALEUCA DAILY FOR LIFE TOTAL NUTRITION FOR WOMEN	US	2
MELALEUCA VITALITY PACK WITH CELLWISE AND PROVEXCV FOR MEN	US	2
MELALEUCA VITALITY PACK WITH CELLWISE AND PROVEXCV FOR WOMEN	US	1½
MEMBER'S MARK DAILY VITAMIN PACK	US	1½
METAGENICS WELLNESS ESSENTIALS	US	4
METAGENICS WELLNESS ESSENTIALS FOR WOMEN	US	3½
MOUNTAIN HOME DAILY ADVANTAGE	US	4½
NATURE MADE DIABETES HEALTH PACK	US	1½
NATURE MADE MAXIMIN PACK	US	2
NATURE MADE MEN'S PACK	US	1
NATURE MADE STRESS PACK	US	1½
NATURE MADE WOMEN'S PACK	US	1
NATURE'S BEST PERFECT FITNESS PAK	US	1½
NATURE'S BEST PERFECT HARDCORE PAK	US	2½
NATURE'S BEST PERFECT SUPER MULTI POWER PAK	US	2½
NATURE'S BOUNTY PRESCRIPTIVE FORMULAS MEN'S	US	1
NATURE'S BOUNTY PRESCRIPTIVE FORMULAS WOMEN'S	US	1½
NATURE'S CODE MEN'S OVER 50	US	2
NATURE'S CODE MEN'S UNDER 50	US	1½

COMBINATION Product Name	Country	# of Stars
Nature's Code Women's Over 50	US	1½
Nature's Code Women's Under 50	US	1½
Nature's Life Mega Pak	US	3
Nature's Peak Fresh Start	CA	2
Nature's Peak Great Start	CA	1½
New Vision Men's Essentials Pack	US	1½
New Vision Prime Pack	US	1½
New Vision Women's Essentials Pack (Coral Calcium)	US	1½
New Vision Women's Essentials Pack (Essential Calcium)	US	2
Nikken Kenzen Dansei/men	US/CA	2½
Nikken Kenzen Josei/women	US/CA	2½
Nsi (Neutraceutical Sciences Institute) Synergy Advanced	US	4½
Nsi (Neutraceutical Sciences Institute) Synergy Max	US	5
Nsi (Neutraceutical Sciences Institute) Synergy Ultra	US	5
Nutricology Super Immuno Complex	US	3
Nutrilite Double X	CA/US	2½
Nutrilite Perfect Health Pack	US	4
Nutristart Nutri-pods	CA	3
Nutrition Dynamics Busy Dad Pack	US	2½
Nutrition Dynamics Busy Mom Pack	US	1
Nutrition Dynamics Cholestavita Forte Pack	US	3
Nutrition Dynamics Just For Dad	US	4½
Nutrivene-d Complete Program	US	2½
Olay Vitamins Daily Energy Pack For Women	US	1
Olay Vitamins Total Effects Beautiful Skin & Wellness	US	2
Olay Vitamins Total Effects Beautiful Skin & Wellness 7x	US	1½
Ortho Molecular Products Alpha Base Foundation Pak	US	4½
Ortho Molecular Products Alpha Base Ultimate Pak	US	5
Pharmanex Lifepak	CA	3½
Pharmanex Lifepak	US	3
Pharmanex Lifepak Nano	CA/US	4
Pharmanex Lifepak Prime	US	3½
Pharmanex Lifepak Women	CA	3
Pharmanex Lifepak Women	US	3
Pharmax Four Pillar Pack	US	2½
Prescriptive Formulas Men's Optimal Vitamin Packs	US	1½
Prescriptive Formulas Women's Optimal Vitamin Packs	US	1½
Pro-caps Laboratories Complete For Men	US	3
Pro-caps Laboratories Complete For Women	US	3½
Pro-caps Laboratories Men's Complete Life Rx	US	3½
Pro-caps Laboratories Men's Maximum Complete	US	3½
Pro-caps Laboratories Ultimate Complete For Men	US	4
Pro-caps Laboratories Ultimate Complete For Women	US	4½
Propax With Nt Factor	US	4
R Garden Essential Nutrition Pack	US	3
R-garden Essential Nutrition Plus	US	3
Safeway Select Maximum Daily Pack	US	2
Safeway Select Men's Daily Pack	US	1
Safeway Select Women's Daily Pack	US	1
Schiff Multi-nutrient Pack	US	2½

COMBINATION Product Name		COUNTRY	# OF STARS
SHAKLEE BASICS IRON FORMULA		US	2½
SHAKLEE BASICS WITH IRON		CA	2
SHAKLEE BASICS WITHOUT IRON		CA	2½
SHAKLEE BASICS WITHOUT IRON		US	2½
SOMALIFE SOMALIFEPAK		US	2½
SOMALIFE SOMALIFEPAK C		CA	2½
SUNDOWN VITAMINS TO GO MAXIMUM		US	1½
SUNDOWN VITAMINS TO GO MEN		US	1
SUNDOWN VITAMINS TO GO WOMEN		US	1
SYMMETRY ULTRA VITALITY NUTRAPACK		US	1½
TOTAL HIGH POTENCY DAILY VITAMIN PACK		US	1
TRIVITA HEALTHY AGING PACK WITH B-12		US	2½
TRIVITA HEALTHY AGING PACK WITH HCY GUARD		US	2½
TRUESTAR HEALTH TRUEBASICS PLUS FOR MEN		CA	5 GOLD
TRUESTAR HEALTH TRUEBASICS PLUS FOR WOMEN		CA	5 GOLD
UNIVERSAL NUTRITION ANIMAL PAK		US	2
UNIVERSAL NUTRITION SPA PAK		US	2
USANA HEALTH SCIENCES HEALTHPAK 100	*EDITOR'S CHOICE*	CA	5 GOLD
USANA HEALTH SCIENCES HEALTHPAK 100	*AWARD WINNERS*	US	5 GOLD
VISALUS VI-PAK		US	4½
VISION FOR LIFE BODY FORCE TRAVEL PACKS		US	2
VITAMIN SHOPPE HEALTH & FITNESS		US	2½
VITAMIN SHOPPE MATURE FEMALE		US	2
VITAMIN SHOPPE MATURE MALE PACK		US	2
VITAMIN SHOPPE MULTI-VITAMIN PACK		US	3
WEIL COMPLETE DAILY PACK		CA	3
WEIL COMPLETE DAILY PACK		US	3
WHEATIES DAILY PERFORMANCE VITAMIN PACK		US	½
XYMOGEN ACTIV ESSENTIALS		US	2
XYMOGEN ACTIV ESSENTIALS WOMEN		US	2
YOURLIFE DAILY PAK MAXIMUM		US	1½
YOURLIFE DAILY PAK MEN'S 50+		US	1½
YOURLIFE DAILY PAK WOMEN'S 50+		US	1